Polypharmacy and Inappropriate Medication Use

Edited by Farid Badria

Published in London, United Kingdom

Polypharmacy and Inappropriate Medication Use
http://dx.doi.org/10.5772/intechopen.1009731
Edited by Farid Badria

Contributors
Abdullah A. Elgazar, Ahmet Çakır, Alfredo Briones-Aranda, Alfredo Vannacci, Costanza Cacini, Farid A. Badria, Giada Crescioli, Hasan Memiş, Roberto Bonaiuti

First published in London, United Kingdom, 2026 by IntechOpen
IntechOpen is the global imprint of INTECHOPEN LIMITED, registered in England and Wales, registration number: 11086078, 167-169 Great Portland Street, London, W1W 5PF, United Kingdom

For EU product safety concerns: IN TECH d.o.o., Prolaz Marije Krucifikse Kozulić 3, 51000 Rijeka, Croatia, info@intechopen.com or visit our website at intechopen.com.

British Library Cataloguing-in-Publication Data
A catalogue record for this book is available from the British Library

Polypharmacy and Inappropriate Medication Use
Edited by Farid Badria
p. cm.

This title is part of the Pharmaceutical Science Book Series, Volume 18
Topic: Pharmacology
Series Editor: Rosario Pignatello
Topic Editor: Cristina Manuela Drăgoi
Associate Topic Editor: Alina Crenguţa Nicolae

Print ISBN 978-1-83635-647-9
Online ISBN 978-1-83635-646-2
eBook (PDF) ISBN 978-1-83635-648-6
ISSN 3033-3318

If disposing of this product, please recycle the paper responsibly.

IntechOpen Book Series
Pharmaceutical Science
Volume 18

Aims and Scope of the Series

Pharmaceutical science focuses on the design, synthesis, formulation, targeting, distribution, safety, and efficacy of active compounds as potential therapeutics. It is a large interdisciplinary discipline that aims to integrate the basic principles of physical and organic chemistry, biochemistry, biology, and engineering to discover, develop, and characterize active compounds and to optimize the formulation and delivery of drugs in the body for offering new and improved safe and efficacious therapies against human diseases. The research areas covered by the pharmaceutical sciences range from medicinal chemistry and pharmaceutical technology to pharmacology and toxicology, which represent the preliminary phases of drug development. Medicinal chemistry involves the design and synthesis of pharmaceuticals as well as the isolation of active agents from natural sources. Computer-aided strategies are increasingly involved in this drug discovery process. Pharmaceutics is a multidisciplinary science that examines the relationships between drug formulation, delivery, distribution, and clinical outcomes. Modern clinical approaches are increasingly relying on controlled release strategies and drug delivery and targeting systems, including nanotechnological platforms (nanomedicine). Pharmacology is the science of drug action in biological systems. Pharmacologists also make drugs as tools to explore aspects of cell and tissue functions. Toxicology is the study of the adverse effects of active agents on living organisms and the ecosystem, including the prevention and amelioration of such adverse effects. This book series includes volumes on Drug Discovery, Delivery, and Pharmacology. Their overall aim is to present the latest research in the whole path of drug discovery and development from different points of view of this multidisciplinary and dynamic field.

Meet the Series Editor

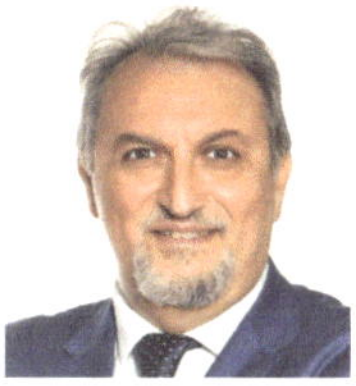

Prof. Rosario Pignatello is a Full Professor of Pharmaceutical Technology and Legislation at the University of Catania, Italy. He is the Director of the Department of Drug and Health Sciences. He has nearly 30 years of experience in the research and development of innovative formulations for the controlled release and targeting of bioactive molecules, through chemical approaches as well as nanotechnological carriers, aimed at treating different disorders. Prof. Pignatello has coauthored about 180 papers and edited a series of textbooks on biomaterials and their application in medicine. The main areas of his research are polymeric and lipid-based micro- and nanoparticles as modified drug delivery systems; vesicular nanocarriers (liposomes, micelles); lipophilic prodrugs and conjugates; synthesis and evaluation of new polymeric biomaterials for drug delivery and tissue regeneration. In particular, Prof. Pignatello works actively in the field of ocular drug delivery, leading the Research Centre for Ocular Nanotechnology, within the NANOMED Centre (Centre for Nanomedicine and Pharmaceutical Nanotechnology) at the University of Catania.

Meet the Volume Editor

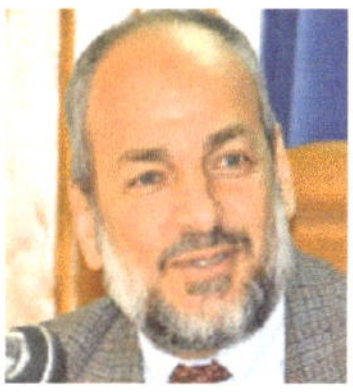

Farid A. Badria is Professor of Pharmacognosy at the Faculty of Pharmacy, Mansoura University, Egypt. He holds a Ph.D. from the University of Minnesota and two M.Sc. degrees from Mansoura and the University of Minnesota. He is the founder and director of FAB-Lab, a natural-product drug discovery lab. His awards include the TWAS Prize for Public Understanding of Science, the WIPO Gold Medal, the State Outstanding Award in Medicine, the Outstanding Arab Scholar Award, and the Khawrazmi International Award. Professor Badria has submitted 47 patent applications, authored over 250 publications and 12 books, and continues to lead research on therapies for liver disease, skin disorders, and cancer.

Contents

Preface

The increasing complexity of healthcare, coupled with the growing burden of chronic diseases and population aging, has made polypharmacy one of the most important contemporary challenges in clinical practice. While the appropriate use of multiple medications may be necessary and beneficial in many patients, especially older adults and individuals with multimorbidity, inappropriate polypharmacy can lead to serious consequences, including adverse drug reactions, drug–drug interactions, poor adherence, reduced quality of life, avoidable hospitalization, and increased healthcare costs.

Polypharmacy and inappropriate medication use represent not only pharmacological concerns but also clinical, ethical, economic, and societal issues. The challenge lies not merely in counting the number of medications a patient receives, but in critically evaluating whether each medication is appropriate, necessary, safe, and aligned with the patient's goals of care. In this context, deprescribing, comprehensive medication management, personalized medicine, and the integration of artificial intelligence into healthcare decision-making have emerged as valuable strategies to optimize therapeutic outcomes and reduce medication-related harm.

This edited volume aims to provide a comprehensive and multidisciplinary overview of the current concepts, challenges, and future directions related to polypharmacy and inappropriate medication use. It brings together contributions from experts in pharmacy, medicine, geriatrics, clinical pharmacology, nursing, healthcare policy, and digital health, reflecting the multifaceted nature of this important issue.

The opening chapters introduce the fundamental definitions, epidemiology, and determinants of polypharmacy, with particular attention to aging populations, multimorbidity, and vulnerable patient groups. These chapters provide readers with an understanding of the scope of the problem and the reasons why polypharmacy has become increasingly prevalent in both developed and developing healthcare systems.

Subsequent chapters explore the clinical consequences of inappropriate medication use, including adverse drug reactions, prescribing cascades, medication errors, drug–drug interactions, and medication non-adherence. Particular emphasis is placed on high-risk populations such as older adults, patients with cognitive impairment, individuals with renal or hepatic dysfunction, and those with chronic cardiovascular, metabolic, psychiatric, or oncological diseases.

The volume also examines validated tools and criteria for assessing medication appropriateness, including medication review frameworks, deprescribing protocols, explicit and implicit prescribing criteria, and risk assessment instruments. These chapters provide practical guidance for healthcare professionals seeking to identify potentially inappropriate medications and improve the safety and effectiveness of pharmacotherapy.

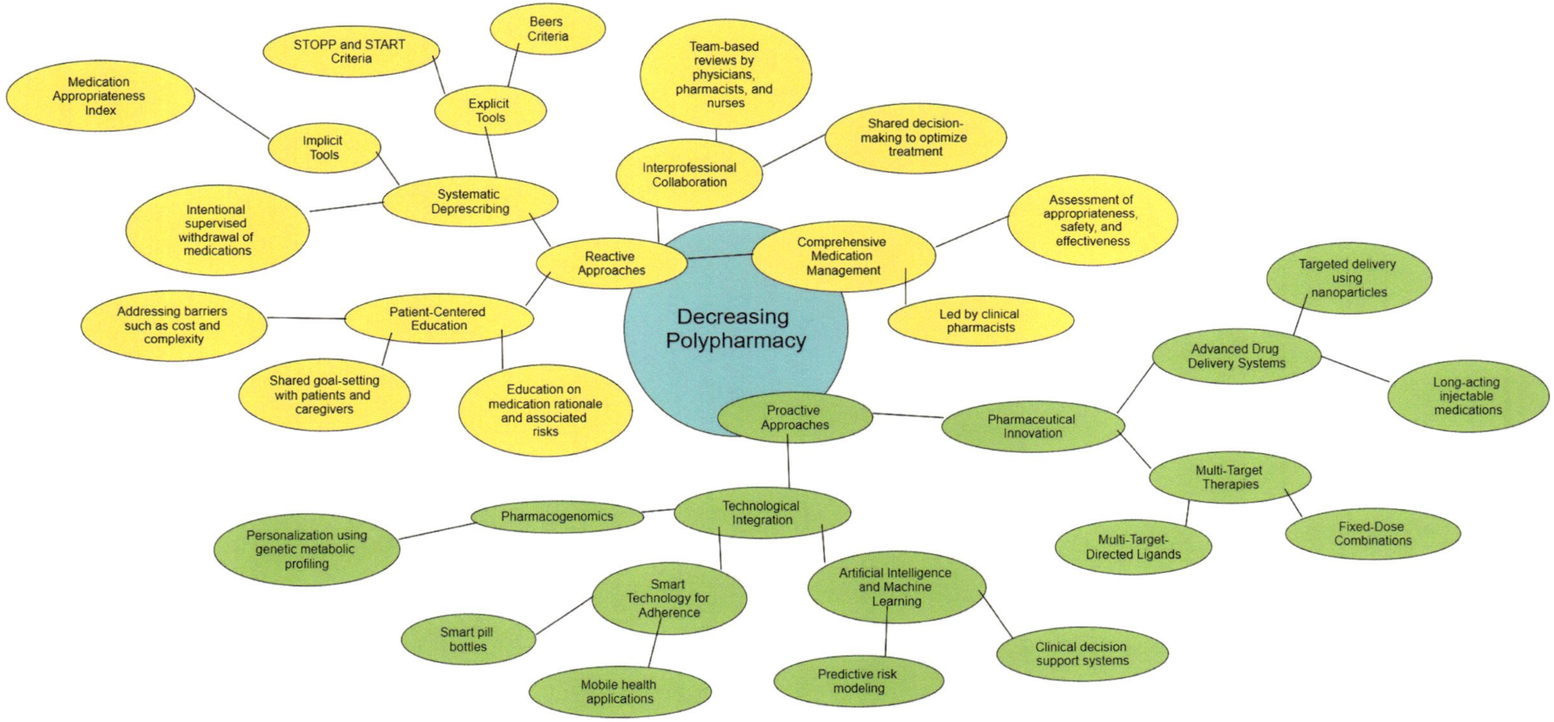

Figure 1.
Presentation of ntegrated approaches to reducing inappropriate polypharmacy. Yellow nodes represent clinical and organizational interventions focused on pharmacotherapy vigilance. Green nodes denote proactive strategies

Special attention is devoted to the role of pharmacists and multidisciplinary healthcare teams in preventing medication-related problems. The contributions highlight the importance of collaborative care, patient counseling, medication reconciliation, and comprehensive medication management in improving therapeutic outcomes and enhancing patient safety.

Recognizing the rapid evolution of healthcare technologies, several chapters address the emerging role of digital health, clinical decision support systems, electronic prescribing, pharmacogenomics, and artificial intelligence in optimizing medication use. These technologies offer promising opportunities to improve prescribing accuracy, reduce preventable harm, and support more individualized therapeutic decisions.

Finally, the concluding chapters discuss future perspectives, policy implications, and recommendations for practice, education, and research. They emphasize the need for stronger interdisciplinary collaboration, better healthcare policies, improved patient medication literacy, and the development of innovative tools to support rational prescribing and deprescribing.

This book is intended for clinicians, pharmacists, nurses, researchers, healthcare administrators, educators, and policymakers who are involved in medication use and patient care. We hope that the chapters presented in this volume will contribute to a deeper understanding of polypharmacy and inappropriate medication use (as shown in **Figure 1**), while also encouraging practical solutions that enhance patient safety, therapeutic effectiveness, and quality of life.

As Academic Editor, I would like to express my sincere gratitude to all chapter authors, reviewers, and editorial staff for their expertise, dedication, and collaborative spirit, which made this volume possible. Their valuable contributions have enriched this book and strengthened its scientific and practical relevance.

Farid A. Badria, Ph.D.D.Sc.
Faculty of Pharmacy,
Pharmacognosy Department,
Mansoura University,
Mansoura, Egypt

Chapter 1

Polypharmacy with Multi-Mechanism Drugs: A Hidden Risk for Drug Interactions and Adverse Effects

Alfredo Briones-Aranda

Abstract

Drugs may overlap in their pharmacokinetic and pharmacodynamic processes, including absorption, distribution, biotransformation, excretion, and mechanism of action. Such overlaps increase the likelihood of interactions as the number of prescribed drugs increases. As a result, polypharmacy carries a significant risk of adverse effects, particularly in older adults. This chapter focuses on drugs such as biguanides, statins, and selective serotonin reuptake inhibitors that act through multiple mechanisms (*polypharmacology*) and may interact directly or indirectly with the serotonergic system, present in the gastrointestinal tract, platelets, and the central nervous system. A clearer understanding of interactions between drugs that share similar targets (*hidden polypharmacy*) can improve knowledge of the pathophysiology underlying adverse drug reactions, and this insight may also be applied to prevent such interactions.

Keywords: polypharmacy, *Polypharmacology*, drug-drug interactions, older adults, oral hypoglycemics, statins, selective serotonin reuptake inhibitors, serotonergic system

1. Introduction

Advances in technology worldwide have driven exponential growth in medical research, resulting in the significant improvements in human health. This progress has contributed to demographic and epidemiological shifts associated with longer life expectancy. Consequently, population aging—now affecting most countries—has become a critical issue and a major challenge for health systems worldwide [1].

Why do aging and the rise of multiple health problems occur together? Aging is well known to bring about a range of physiological changes and is closely associated with a higher prevalence of chronic degenerative diseases (CDDs), including type 2 diabetes mellitus (T2DM), as well as cardiovascular, renal, and rheumatologic conditions, among others [2, 3].

In this complex context, multi- and interdisciplinary medical care is essential, with daily clinical collaboration providing common ground for specialists such as internists, cardiologists, and geriatricians, as well as other health professionals including nurses, gerontologists, nutritionists, psychologists, and physiotherapists. When faced with frailty and CDDs, these professionals may prescribe multiple pharmacological treatments alongside self-care measures, such as promoting physical activity and adopting hygienic-dietary strategies, all aimed at helping patients cope and maintain homeostasis.

Polypharmacy is generally defined as the use of five or more medications [4], which may be potentially inappropriate [4, 5] or unnecessary [6]. Its prevalence is particularly high among older adults: It is estimated that more than 50% take five or more drugs, and over 10% take 10 or more [7], greatly increasing risks to their health and overall well-being [8]. According to a WHO report published in 2019, polypharmacy is a major and growing public health problem across healthcare settings worldwide [9].

As noted above, drugs may overlap in their pharmacokinetic processes—absorption, distribution, biotransformation, and excretion—and may also share similarities in their mechanisms of action. Such overlaps can lead to drug-drug interactions (DDIs), with the number of prescribed medications being a major contributing factor [10, 11].

The clinical outcomes of DDIs can range from diminished to enhanced effects of one or more drugs, with the latter often manifesting as adverse drug reactions (ADRs) [12].

However, the emergence of multi-mechanism drugs—agents that act on multiple targets simultaneously (pleiotropic)—has introduced new challenges. These drugs were initially designed to improve efficacy but also add hidden risks of interaction. Some can initiate biochemical changes that directly or indirectly trigger cascades of additional effects, impacting multiple systems. In line with this, most drugs used in the treatment of oncological [13] or psychiatric [14] disorders are characterized by multiple mechanisms of action (*polypharmacology*). For example, clozapine, used as an antipsychotic, can interact with several neurotransmission systems, including dopaminergic, serotonergic, muscarinic, and histaminergic pathways [15]. Similarly, tyrosine kinase inhibitors can block various enzymes that cancer cells rely on to grow and divide rapidly [16]. Nevertheless, other drugs with this same characteristic—such as oral hypoglycemics (78%) and statins (62%)—are of particular importance due to their frequent prescription as part of polypharmacy in studies involving geriatric populations [17].

In consideration of the above, the primary purpose of this chapter is to explore the risks of DDIs and ADRs associated with hidden polypharmacy involving drugs with polypharmacology, such as oral hypoglycemics, statins, and selective serotonin reuptake inhibitors (SSRIs). This analysis draws on experimental and clinical research with the aim of proposing strategies for the responsible prescription of these medications in adults over 65 years of age with CDDs.

Because polypharmacy in the geriatric population can negatively affect health—ranging from an increased risk of DDIs to the onset of adverse effects such as cognitive decline [18], cataracts [19], and malnutrition [20]—it also contributes to poor treatment adherence [6] and increased hospitalizations caused by ADRs [21]. These consequences are closely linked to greater frailty and higher healthcare costs [6].

2. Physiological changes associated with aging that may influence pharmacokinetic processes

2.1 General considerations

The world is undergoing a major demographic shift. By 2050, the number of people over 60 years of age is expected to rise from 600 million to nearly 2 billion, with the fastest and largest growth occurring in developing countries, where the elderly population is projected to quadruple over the next 50 years [22]. Aging has been defined in many ways, but a comprehensive perspective describes it as a process involving morphological, functional, and psychological changes that alter the structure and function of different systems, increasing an individual's vulnerability to environmental stress and disease [23]. However, the pace of these changes varies across organs and systems, as well as among individuals. Aging is also characterized by alterations in the phases of pharmacokinetic processes, which may affect the bioavailability and therapeutic effectiveness of prescribed drugs [24].

On the other hand, it is necessary to revisit two closely related terms that could cause confusion: *polypharmacology* and *polypharmacy* (**Figure 1**). The former refers to molecules that can interact with multiple molecular targets [25], while the latter, defined earlier, has two dimensions. Traditional polypharmacy refers to the prescription and administration of several potentially inappropriate drugs that may interact primarily at the pharmacokinetic level, such as through shared metabolism (**Figure 1**). In contrast, *hidden polypharmacy* may refer to the use of a drug with polypharmacology, which can lead to complex problematic interactions at both the pharmacokinetic and pharmacodynamic levels [25, 26], since multiple actions of a single drug may provoke the adverse effects comparable to those observed with

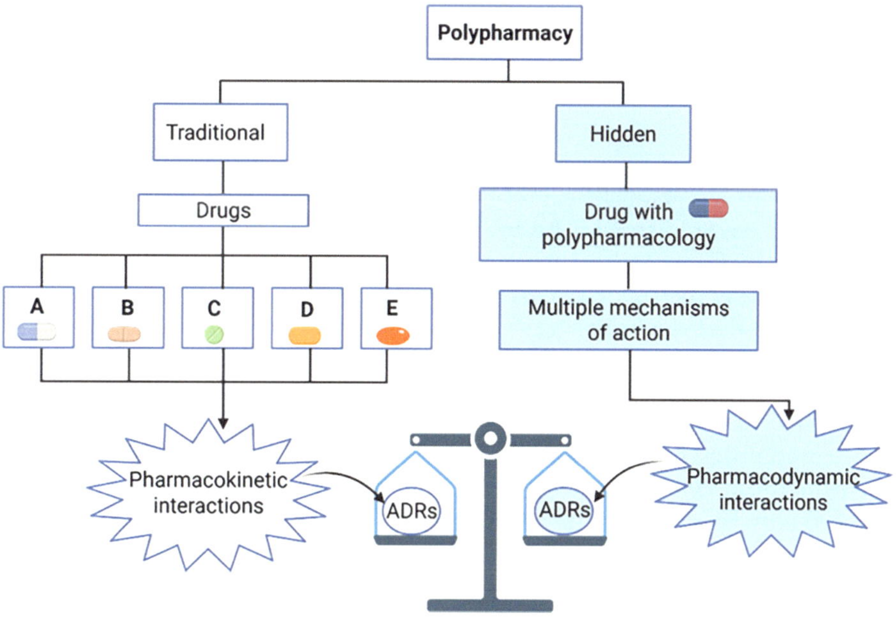

Figure 1.
Differences and similarities between traditional and hidden polypharmacy. Created with https://BioRender.com.

traditional polypharmacy (**Figure 1**). However, the term *hidden polypharmacy* may also apply when herbal medicines or dietary supplements are combined with the standard treatments, a practice frequently observed among geriatric patients and often not reported to their treating physicians [27].

Therefore, before addressing the potential interactions of drugs with polypharmacology, it is necessary to establish a theoretical framework concerning the physiological changes that occur during aging and strongly influence pharmacokinetic processes.

Figure 1 shows that traditional polypharmacy, which consists of the administration of five or more drugs, may involve interactions at the pharmacokinetic level and trigger adverse drug reactions (ADRs). By contrast, in hidden polypharmacy, a single drug with multiple mechanisms of action (polypharmacology) can interact at the pharmacodynamic level and produce equivalent ADRs.

2.2 Oral absorption

Evidence on age-related changes in gastric secretion is inconsistent. Some studies report that gastric acid secretion does not significantly decline in healthy older adults [28, 29], while others suggest it may even increase [30]. In addition, cases of achlorhydria and hypochlorhydria have been documented in this population [31, 32]. Such changes can directly affect drug solubility and gastric emptying. It is well established that higher gastric acidity reduces the dissociation of acidic drugs, and their lower polarity in this state favors absorption. By contrast, weakly basic drugs (e.g., ketoconazole, ampicillin, and iron supplements) dissociate more readily in an acidic pH, which limits their absorption. In hypochlorhydria, the reduced acidity may impair the dissociation and absorption of weakly basic drugs such as ketoconazole [33].

Most studies on age-related gastric emptying report that it is delayed and reduced in older adults. This slowing is generally associated with decreased appetite and impaired absorption of both nutrients and drugs [34].

2.3 Distribution

Total body water remains stable compared with that of young adults until about age 60, after which it gradually declines [35]. This reduction is thought to result mainly from a loss of intracellular water, as extracellular water remains stable. These changes directly affect highly water-soluble drugs such as acetaminophen: A smaller apparent volume of distribution (Vd) leads to faster rises in plasma concentrations after administration, underscoring the need for initial dose adjustments [36].

In contrast, adipose tissue tends to increase from about age 30 onward, which can expand the Vd of lipophilic drugs such as benzodiazepines [37, 38]. This results in lower plasma concentrations and greater drug accumulation in fat tissue, contributing to redistribution and prolongation of half-life.

Drug binding to plasma proteins is also influenced by age. In healthy older adults, plasma albumin levels may decline by up to 30% compared with younger adults, causing drugs that bind strongly to this protein to exhibit the increased pharmacological activity [39, 40]. These effects are even more pronounced in pathological conditions such as chronic malnutrition and renal failure, where plasma protein levels may be significantly reduced [41].

One of the most widely studied effects of aging is the decline in cardiac output, which leads to reduced circulating volume, increased vascular resistance, and microcirculatory changes. These alterations limit the body's ability to distribute drugs efficiently and may affect the Vd [42]. Notably, the hepatic and renal vascular networks are among the most impacted by reduced blood flow in older adults [43].

2.4 Metabolism

In older adults, physiological changes such as reduced liver mass, decreased hepatic blood flow, and diminished metabolic capacity alter drug metabolism. These factors play a key role in the decline of first-pass metabolism often seen in geriatric patients [42, 43]. As a result, the bioavailability of certain drugs, such as propranolol, may rise significantly, requiring lower initial doses [44, 45]. Conversely, reduced first-pass metabolism can hinder the activation of several prodrugs, including angiotensin-converting enzyme inhibitors like enalapril, potentially leading to lower systemic levels of the active compound [46].

Overall, the decline in hepatic metabolism in older adults varies by drug and by individual. Age-related changes mainly affect phase I metabolism (oxidation, reduction, and hydrolysis), whereas phase II metabolism (glucuronidation, acetylation, and sulfation) is generally less impacted [47, 48].

In addition, the hepatic and intestinal enzyme CYP3A4 is the most abundant, and approximately 50% of marketed drugs are metabolized through this pathway [49]. This enzyme is particularly relevant for drugs that act as substrates, inducers, or inhibitors. Of special concern is the combination of CYP3A4-inhibiting drugs with pleiotropic drugs that behave as substrates [50]—for example, a macrolide administered together with a statin, a scenario discussed later in this chapter.

Another important consideration involves psychiatric [51] and oncological [52] patient populations, who are often treated with polypharmacy regimens. In these cases, combinations such as the chemotherapeutic agent cyclosporine together with a CYP3A4 inhibitor like the antifungal itraconazole can trigger toxic effects [53].

Finally, another key factor is the presence of polymorphisms associated with the CYP2D6 gene, which reduces hepatic biotransformation and affects the metabolism of various drugs, including antidepressants, antipsychotics, opioid analgesics, beta-blockers, and antiarrhythmics. Such alterations may promote drug accumulation and consequently increase the risk of ADRs [54].

2.5 Elimination

In older adults, physiological changes that can affect renal drug elimination include reduced renal blood flow, decreased glomerular filtration, and diminished tubular secretory capacity [55, 56]. Renal function is commonly assessed using the pharmacokinetic parameter clearance, which depends on creatinine elimination. Creatinine clearance declines by about one-third between ages 20 and 90, although the rate of decline varies among individuals [57, 58].

Reduced glomerular filtration and tubular function are the main factors limiting the clearance of many drugs, including water-soluble antibiotics, diuretics, digoxin, beta-blockers, lithium, and nonsteroidal anti-inflammatory drugs (NSAIDs) [55, 59, 60]. In addition, the combined administration of angiotensin-converting enzyme inhibitors (ACEIs), NSAIDs, and diuretics can reduce both renal blood flow and glomerular filtration, thereby enhancing nephrotoxicity [61]. These effects are further aggravated by common comorbidities in older adults, such as T2DM and hypertension [58, 62].

The clinical significance of reduced renal excretion in older adults lies in its potential to cause adverse drug reactions (ADRs) or drug toxicity. For medications with a narrow therapeutic index, such as aminoglycoside antibiotics [63], digoxin, and lithium [64], even slight accumulation can result in serious ADRs [56, 65]. Thus, impaired renal function in older adults must be carefully considered to avoid overdosing.

3. Examples of drugs with multiple mechanisms of action that may increase the risk of interactions and ADRs in the geriatric population

3.1 Oral hypoglycemics

3.1.1 Pharmacokinetics of biguanides

Among this group, metformin is the most widely used drug for the treatment of T2DM. It is absorbed in the small intestine with an approximate bioavailability of 50–60% [66]. Metformin shows minimal binding to plasma proteins, is not metabolized in the liver, and is not excreted in bile. Instead, it is eliminated almost entirely by the kidneys, primarily through active tubular secretion [67]. Currently, there is no strong clinical evidence of pharmacokinetic DDIs involving metformin.

3.1.2 Importance of the multiple effects of metformin and their possible implications for adverse drug reactions

Metformin is considered a drug with polypharmacological properties, as it can act on multiple regions of the body, including the gastrointestinal system, liver, pancreas, and skeletal muscle [68]. In older adults, significant delays in gastric emptying may occur, potentially affecting the intestinal absorption of metformin. The main transporters involved in its absorption and intestinal transport include: a) organic cation transporter 1 (OCT-1), b) plasma membrane monoamine transporter (PMAT), and c) serotonin transporter (SERT), among others [69, 70]. Because much of this evidence comes from animal studies, further research in humans is needed (**Figure 1**).

OCT-1 can be inhibited by proton pump inhibitors (PPIs) such as pantoprazole [71], which may reduce metformin absorption and, in turn, lower its hypoglycemic effect [72]. Moreover, combining these drugs can lead to gastrointestinal side effects, including diarrhea and abdominal discomfort [73].

In the intestine, metformin can also reduce glucose absorption [74] and impair the absorption of vitamin B12 and bile acids [75, 76]. Gastrointestinal intolerance is a well-recognized syndrome associated with metformin. Diarrhea is among the most common clinical manifestations [75, 77], although other studies have identified nausea and vomiting as the additional major adverse effects [78, 79].

One proposed mechanism for gastrointestinal intolerance involves the GLP-1 receptor [79]. Another theory suggests that metformin may alter intestinal 5-HT levels, triggering diarrhea, nausea, and vomiting similar to metformin intolerance [80]. Metformin also has structural similarities to selective 5-HT3 receptor agonists [81], which acts on receptors that regulate nausea and vomiting [80]. However, some studies have found no consistent evidence linking metformin-induced nausea to interactions with this receptor [80, 81].

Interestingly, metformin may also interact with other serotonergic receptor subtypes, such as 5-HT1A and 5-HT1B. In previous studies, the antagonists WAY-100635 and GR-127935—specific blockers of the 5-HT1A and 5-HT1B receptors, respectively—were found to inhibit the antinociceptive effects of metformin [82]. In addition, stimulation of the 5-HT2C receptor can enhance 5-HT release from the duodenum [83].

Gluconeogenesis is the metabolic process of producing glucose from non-carbohydrate precursors such as lactate, glycerol, and certain amino acids. It plays a key role in maintaining normal blood glucose levels, particularly during fasting or when glycogen stores are depleted. Metformin inhibits gluconeogenesis, thereby lowering blood glucose. It also acts on the mitochondrial respiratory chain by inhibiting Complex I [84]. Consequently, by limiting the liver's ability to convert lactate into glucose, metformin may increase the blood lactate levels.

Although metformin is considered safe for most patients with T2DM, in certain situations it may increase the risk of lactic acidosis, particularly when combined with drugs that impair its renal clearance, disrupt acid–base balance, or alter lactate metabolism [85].

Medications such as NSAIDs, angiotensin-converting enzyme inhibitors, and angiotensin II receptor antagonists can acutely reduce glomerular filtration, leading to metformin accumulation and an increased risk of lactic acidosis, particularly in the setting of dehydration or hypovolemia [85–87]. Additional risk factors include excessive alcohol consumption, high doses of metformin combined with prolonged fasting, intense physical exercise, renal impairment, severe infections, and carbon dioxide poisoning, all of which can further raise the likelihood of lactic acidosis [88, 89].

T2DM is characterized by impairments in both insulin secretion and insulin sensitivity [90]. Insulin release from pancreatic β-cells plays a central role in the disease's etiology, but the complex regulation and mechanisms by which metformin influences β-cell insulin secretion are not yet fully understood [91]. Evidence suggests that metformin can downregulate the nitric oxide (NO) system in β-cells, which normally acts as a negative regulator of insulin secretion. In experimental models, metformin suppresses NO overproduction induced by high glucose concentrations or sulfonylureas, potentially restoring the insulin secretory response [92, 93].

The 5-HT1B and 5-HT2C receptors also play distinct roles in regulating insulin secretion from pancreatic β-cells [94, 95]. However, studies have shown that activation of the 5-HT1B receptor in humans and the 5-HT2C receptor in mice reduces insulin release (**Figure 1**) [95, 96].

These findings are both intriguing and complex, as the 5-HT1A [97] and 5-HT1B [98] receptors—potential targets of metformin—are not only expressed in β-cells but also located on the platelet plasma membrane, where the 5-HT1B receptor in particular has been associated with platelet aggregation (**Figure 2**) [98, 99].

The GABAergic system has likewise been linked to insulin secretion [100]. Evidence suggests that GABA may promote β-cell proliferation [101], and benzodiazepine receptor agonists have been shown to enhance pancreatic β-cell function (**Figure 2**) [102]. Another noteworthy finding is metformin's potential affinity for the GABAA receptor, reported in preclinical studies, where this biguanide demonstrated the anxiolytic effects through interaction with the GABAA receptor [103].

Additional evidence of the complex interplay between the serotonergic system (SS), the GABAergic system, behavioral disorders, and the metabolic disturbances characteristic of T2DM is the presence of 5-HT1B, 5-HT2C, and GABAA receptors in various regions of the CNS (**Figure 1**), including the raphe nuclei, hippocampus, and

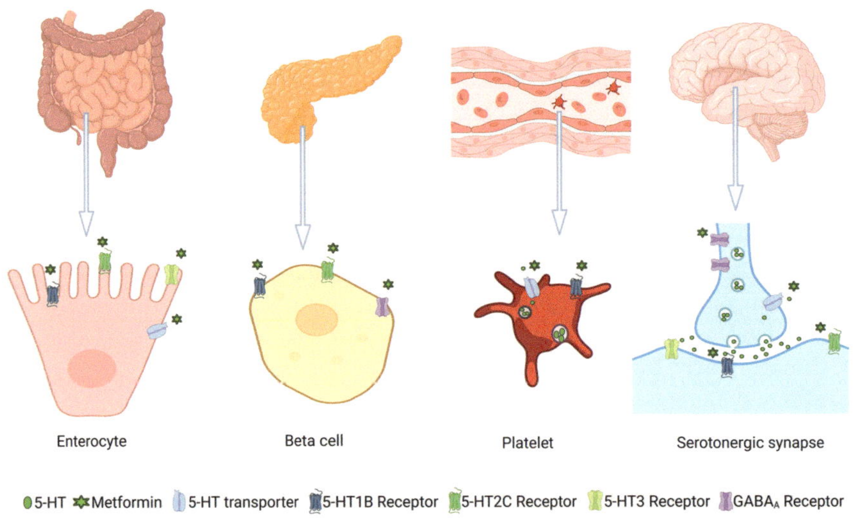

Figure 2.
Possible sites of action of metformin. The diagram illustrates metformin's interactions at the intestinal, pancreatic, vascular, and central nervous system (CNS) levels. In each of these regions, this biguanide may specifically interact with serotonergic and GABAergic receptors, as well as with the serotonin transporter. Created with BioRender.com.

prefrontal cortex—areas involved in memory regulation [104], depression [105], and anxiety [106]. Notably, there is a bidirectional relationship between the metabolic dysfunction associated with T2DM and the prevalence of depression [107].

Metformin's multiple mechanisms of action add a significant layer of complexity to its clinical use, beyond the potential DDIs associated with biguanides. For example, in older adults undergoing polypharmacy, PPIs may be prescribed for acid-peptic disease or SSRIs for depression. Riskier prescriptions, such as benzodiazepines for sleep disorders in diabetic patients treated with metformin, may also be introduced. Another frequent scenario is the use of NSAIDs, such as acetylsalicylic acid, for vascular disease prevention.

Given these situations, physicians should be especially vigilant for ADRs that may appear difficult to explain but could, in fact, be linked to metformin's ability to interact with the serotonergic and GABAergic systems in multiple regions of the body.

3.2 Statins

3.2.1 Pharmacology of statins

Statins are a group of drugs that include lovastatin, pravastatin, simvastatin, fluvastatin, cerivastatin, rosuvastatin, and atorvastatin. Their mechanism of action is based on inhibition of the enzyme 3-hydroxy-3-methylglutaryl-coenzyme A reductase (HMG-CoAR) [108].

Atorvastatin is rapidly absorbed after oral administration, with peak plasma concentrations reached in about 4 hours. Its absolute bioavailability is 12%, and both the rate and extent of absorption are influenced by the time of administration and food intake [109]. Atorvastatin binds to plasma albumin by approximately 98% and has a half-life of roughly 14 to 20 hours [86]. After hepatic metabolism, it is excreted primarily in the bile [110].

Statins are indicated for reducing elevated total cholesterol, low-density lipoprotein cholesterol (LDL-C), very-low-density lipoprotein (VLDL) synthesis, and circulating triglycerides in patients with primary hypercholesterolemia [111]. By improving dyslipidemia, statins reduce the risk of cardiovascular events and mortality [112].

Atorvastatin is mainly metabolized by CYP3A4, which makes it vulnerable to DDIs with enzyme inhibitors such as clarithromycin and erythromycin [113]. In such cases, plasma concentrations of atorvastatin may rise substantially, increasing the risk of adverse effects including myopathy and rhabdomyolysis [114].

Atorvastatin is also a substrate of hepatic transporters, including OATP1B3. Co-administration with cyclosporine, an OATP1B1 inhibitor, can significantly increase its bioavailability [115]. In contrast, CYP3A4 inducers such as rifampicin may reduce plasma concentrations of atorvastatin [116]. Furthermore, combining atorvastatin with fibrates or niacin increases the risk of myopathy and rhabdomyolysis through additive effects on muscle pathways [117, 118].

In addition, statins have been associated with clinically evident cases of acute liver injury, presenting with hepatocellular or cholestatic patterns [119]. Concomitant use with other drugs that carry a risk of hepatotoxicity—such as NSAIDs [120], selective serotonin reuptake inhibitors (SSRIs) [121], amoxicillin-clavulanic acid [122], and anticonvulsants [120]—may potentiate liver damage.

3.2.2 Importance of the multiple effects of atorvastatin and potential adverse drug reactions

It is also important to consider the concomitant effects that may result from atorvastatin-induced cholesterol reduction. Cholesterol is the primary substrate for the synthesis of several steroid hormones [123, 124].

With regard to hormones, some studies have suggested that statins may slightly reduce the synthesis of certain steroids, although results have been inconsistent. Clinical and epidemiological evidence has generally shown no significant effects on the production of cortisol, total or free testosterone, estradiol, LH, or FSH [125–127]. However, in women with polycystic ovary syndrome, statins have been shown to reduce androgen levels and improve hyperandrogenism, although their use for this purpose is not recommended outside of cardiovascular indications [125].

Conflicting evidence has also been reported regarding a possible bidirectional interaction between statins and gonadal hormones. For instance, statin use has been associated with an increased risk of T2DM in postmenopausal women [127, 128], and in this same group, one study found that intensive statin therapy over 1 year did not slow the progression of coronary calcification [129]. Conversely, other studies have suggested that statins do not significantly affect gonadal function or fertility in either men or women, nor do they appear to alter the menstrual cycle or progesterone synthesis in premenopausal women [130, 131]. It is important to note, however, that women have been underrepresented in statin trials, and data on efficacy and safety in this population remain limited.

In light of the above, hormonal status is an important factor that may influence the development of statin-related adverse effects. Further and more in-depth research is needed to account for this variable and to clarify the presence or absence of such potential effects.

Regarding the SS, statins may influence 5-HT neurotransmission through both cholesterol-dependent and cholesterol-independent mechanisms. Experimental studies have shown that chronic cholesterol depletion induced by statins can alter the function and dynamics of 5-HT1A receptors, reducing their coupling to G proteins and their ability to bind ligands. These alterations may help explain the symptoms of anxiety and depression observed in some patients undergoing statin therapy (**Figure 3B**) [132, 133].

Statins have also been shown to enhance 5-HT reuptake through SERT in a fluoxetine-dependent manner, *via* cholesterol-independent lipid signaling pathways, specifically through the regulation of isoprenylation intermediates such as farnesyl pyrophosphate [134]. These effects on the SS have been demonstrated in cell and animal models; however, their clinical significance remains uncertain, as some studies have suggested a possible association between statin use and the development of depression [133].

Statins have been used for nearly four decades, with their effectiveness in treating cardiovascular disease well supported by extensive evidence. Nevertheless, many studies have also linked them to potential adverse effects on mental health.

Preclinical studies have associated statins with cognitive impairment. In male rats, daily oral administration of pravastatin or atorvastatin (10 mg/kg) for 18 days impaired learning during the final days of treatment, an effect that was fully reversed after discontinuation [135]. Likewise, in a novel object recognition task, pravastatin significantly impaired memory.

Furthermore, oral administration of simvastatin at doses of 10 or 30 mg/kg/day in rats for 4 weeks led to impaired spatial memory, as measured by the Barnes maze test [136]. Similarly, in a study with male guinea pigs, the effects of simvastatin (2 mg/kg) and atorvastatin (1 mg/kg, oral) were evaluated over 6 weeks. Spatial memory was tested using the Morris water maze, and animals treated with statins spent significantly more time outside the platform area compared with controls [137].

The memory impairment observed may be explained by several interconnected mechanisms. One key factor is the structural role of cholesterol in neuronal membranes, where it is essential for synapse formation, neurotransmitter release, and the proper function of membrane receptors such as Glu, DA, and 5-HT receptors [138].

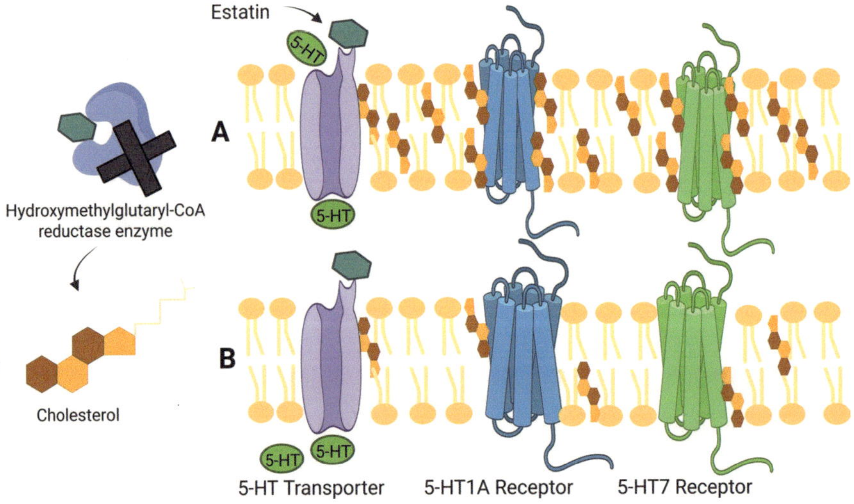

Figure 3.
Influence of statin-induced membrane cholesterol reduction on serotonergic receptors.

Lipophilic statins, such as atorvastatin, can cross the blood-brain barrier and lower brain cholesterol levels. This may impair synaptic plasticity and neuronal transmission, contributing to deficits in spatial and recognition memory [139]. Such effects are linked to reduce membrane fluidity and decreased availability of anchoring sites for receptors such as 5-HT1A and 5-HT7, which depend on intact lipid microdomains for effective signaling [140, 141].

Several studies have also shown that, in certain contexts, atorvastatin can exert proinflammatory effects, increasing cytokines such as IL-1β, TNF-α, and IL-6—particularly in experimental models with prior immune challenges or under hormonal conditions such as estrogen deprivation [142]. The activation of inflammatory pathways may further exacerbate cognitive decline by suppressing neurotrophic factors such as BDNF and impairing neurogenesis in the hippocampus, a region critical for memory consolidation [142].

Panel A illustrates the membrane cholesterol configuration that provides anchoring and stability to the 5-HT1A and 5-HT7 serotonergic receptors, as well as the potential interaction of certain statins with the 5-HT transporter. Panel B depicts the possible impact of statin-induced membrane cholesterol reduction on serotonergic receptors. Created with https://BioRender.com

It is therefore plausible to suggest that the combination of estrogen deficiency and subchronic atorvastatin treatment in animals involves complex mechanisms that may act synergistically to worsen memory impairment. Both factors also affect the SS, as cholesterol depletion [141] and estrogen deficiency [143] have been shown to alter the density and function of serotonergic receptors, including 5-HT1A and 5-HT7R. Such changes directly impact processes such as working memory, consolidation, and spatial learning, which are associated with these receptors (**Figure 3**) [143].

In this context, the convergence of lipid dysfunction, estrogen deficiency, neuroinflammation, and serotonergic disruption may represent key interrelated factors underlying statin-induced cognitive deficits in animal models. Collectively, these findings underscore the complexity of statins' effects on cognitive function.

Finally, although randomized clinical trials and systematic reviews have not demonstrated significant differences in cognitive performance, memory, executive function, or in the incidence of dementia or Alzheimer's disease between statin users and controls [144, 145], it remains important to monitor pharmacovigilance data and pursue further research on these potential cognitive effects. This is especially relevant in women, to better confirm or rule out ADRs and provide greater therapeutic certainty for this widely used drug class in the geriatric population.

3.3 Selective serotonin reuptake inhibitors

3.3.1 Pharmacology of selective serotonin reuptake inhibitors

SSRIs differ by specific compound but share general characteristics important for clinical practice. They have largely replaced tricyclic antidepressants as the first-line treatment for major depressive disorder [146]. In addition, they are indicated for anorexia nervosa, bulimia nervosa, and several anxiety-related disorders [147], including obsessive-compulsive disorder, panic disorder, social phobia, and post-traumatic stress disorder [148].

Furthermore, fluoxetine [149] and other agents such as duloxetine and venlafaxine—classified as serotonin-norepinephrine reuptake inhibitors (SNRIs)—are also widely used as first-line treatments for neuropathic pain [150].

SSRIs (fluoxetine, sertraline, paroxetine, fluvoxamine, citalopram, escitalopram) are well absorbed orally but have moderate bioavailability due to first-pass hepatic metabolism. They are widely distributed in tissues and bind extensively to plasma proteins [147]. Elimination occurs primarily through hepatic cytochrome P450 isoenzymes, resulting in substantial interindividual variability in plasma concentrations and an increased risk of DDIs.

In the CNS, SSRIs alter serotonin (5-hydroxytryptamine, 5-HT) release and reuptake, influencing synaptic plasticity and functional connectivity in brain regions associated with depression, including the anterior cingulate cortex, amygdala, and hippocampus [151–153]. Modulation of 5-HT2C receptor activity can either enhance or counteract SSRI effects on 5-HT release and the antidepressant response, as demonstrated in preclinical studies [154–156].

Fluoxetine and paroxetine are potent CYP2D6 inhibitors, which can elevate plasma concentrations of drugs metabolized through this pathway, including antipsychotics (haloperidol and clozapine), tricyclic antidepressants, and certain beta-blockers.

Consistent with this, a growing number of previous studies have reported that combining SSRIs with newer antipsychotics (e.g., clozapine, olanzapine, risperidone, sertindole, aripiprazole, ziprasidone, quetiapine) in geriatric patients has been associated with cases of arrhythmias, QTc interval prolongation on electrocardiograms, orthostatic hypotension, and confusion [157]. These alterations have, in turn, been linked to an increased risk of falls that may lead to fractures [158].

Fluvoxamine mainly inhibits CYP1A2 and CYP2C19, potentially increasing levels of drugs such as theophylline, warfarin, and several anticonvulsants (**Figure 4**).

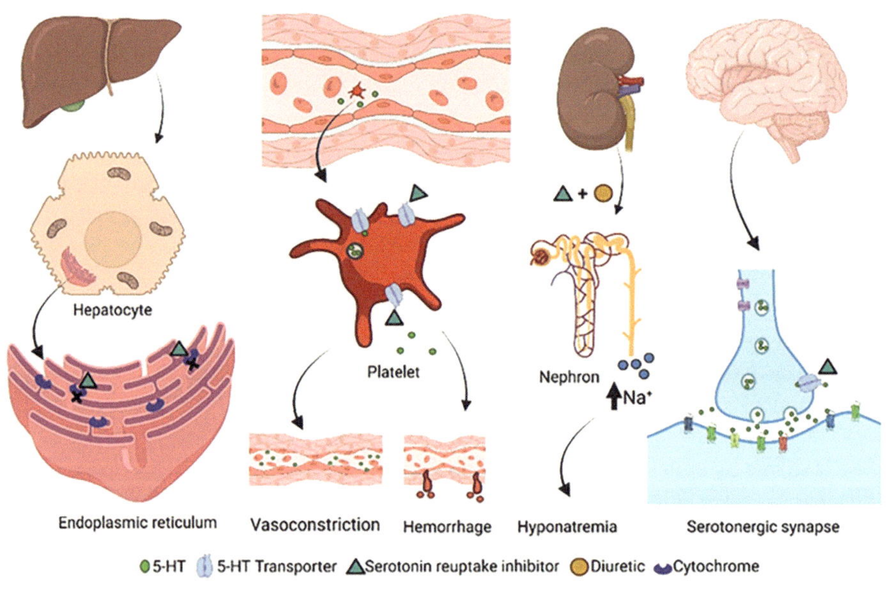

Figure 4.
Multiple effects of SSRIs. The diagram outlines both the pharmacokinetic and pharmacodynamic effects of SSRIs that may explain adverse drug reactions related to interactions at the metabolic, renal, vascular, and central nervous system levels. In the latter two regions, these drugs may alter SS physiology, potentially leading to adverse outcomes such as elevated blood pressure and hemorrhage. Created with https://BioRender.com.

In addition, SSRIs can interact with other neurotransmitter systems. Fluoxetine and paroxetine, for instance, inhibit nicotinic receptors, which may contribute to the neurological side effects and alter cholinergic activity [159].

SSRIs may also increase the risk of upper gastrointestinal bleeding by inhibiting platelet SERT [146, 160]. This risk can be further elevated when they are used in combination with drugs that affect hemostasis, such as NSAIDs or anticoagulants [161, 162].

3.3.2 Importance of the multiple indirect effects of SSRIs and their possible implications for adverse drug reactions

As with the two drug groups discussed above, SSRIs may also have overlapping effects because of their ability to modulate extracellular 5-HT levels. Since the SS is involved in multiple organs and systems, changes in 5-HT concentrations can trigger a wide range of effects and may interact with the mechanisms of action of other drugs.

Although some adverse effects of SSRIs are rare, they are clinically significant due to the sharp rise in their use over recent decades, especially among older adults and patients with T2DM and depression [163]. In addition, serious adverse effects are increasingly being reported, including hyponatremia, bleeding, increased risk of suicidal ideation, and cardiovascular complications with certain SSRIs.

SSRI-induced hyponatremia is defined as a plasma sodium concentration below 136 mEq/L. Symptoms typically appear at levels under 130 mEq/L, with values below 125 mEq/L considered severe. At 125–130 mEq/L, gastrointestinal symptoms are most common, while lower levels are associated with neuropsychiatric manifestations.

Risk factors for hyponatremia include age over 65 years, female sex, concomitant diuretic use, low body weight, and baseline plasma sodium levels near the lower limit of normal before initiating SSRI therapy (**Figure 3**) [164].

SSRI therapy has also been linked to increased reports of hypertension, both as a new-onset condition and as worsening of preexisting hypertension [165]. However, the magnitude of this risk appears to vary among different agents, and no clear dose-response relationship has been established [166].

In terms of cardiovascular safety, certain SSRIs—particularly citalopram and escitalopram—can prolong the QTc interval, a concern especially relevant for patients with heart failure or those at risk of arrhythmias [167, 168].

4. Possible strategies to prevent drug interactions involving multiple mechanisms of action in the geriatric population

The risk of developing DDIs—and consequently ADRs—is well known to increase in proportion to the number of drugs prescribed. The more medications a patient takes, the greater the likelihood of overlapping pharmacokinetic and pharmacodynamic processes.

Beyond these overlaps, special attention should be given to drugs with multiple mechanisms of action, whether direct or indirect, such as biguanides, statins, and SSRIs, which have been discussed above as illustrative examples.

For this reason, physicians must exercise particular caution when prescribing these drugs as part of therapy for older adults.

Since drugs with multiple mechanisms of action add an extra layer of risk to DDIs, they further increase the likelihood of interactions with other medications and, consequently, the exponential probability of developing ADRs.

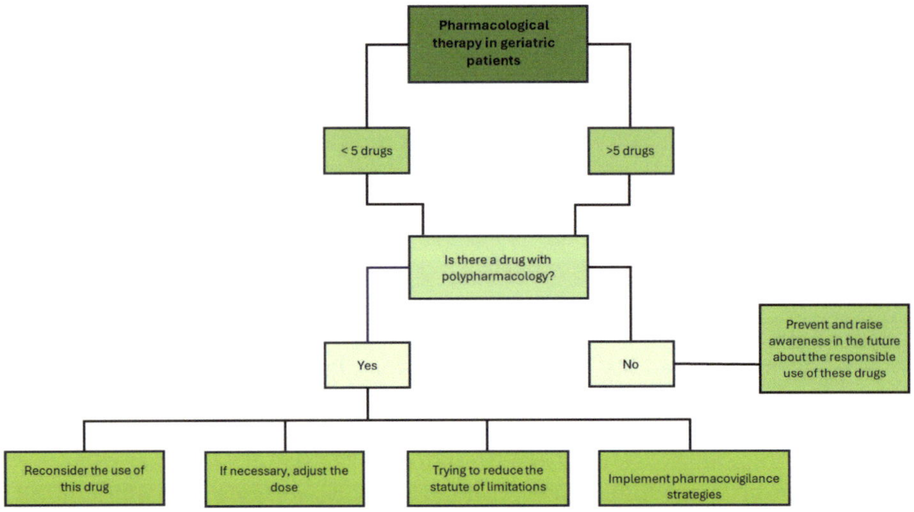

Figure 5.
Algorithm for the management of drugs with multiple mechanisms of action.

Thus, even when fewer than five drugs are prescribed, the presence of a single drug with multiple mechanisms of action should be taken seriously. In such cases, strategies should be implemented to prevent or promptly detect the potential adverse effects.

Building on the discussion above, an algorithm has been developed to provide a clear and practical framework for managing the prescription of drugs with polypharmacology in the geriatric population (**Figure 5**).

When assessing the risk of clinically relevant DDIs in older adults, additional factors should be considered, including multiple prescribers, infrequent or inadequate monitoring, impaired drug elimination pathways, and pharmacogenetic variability. Effective communication between healthcare providers and patients is therefore essential, with treating physicians and nurses playing a central role in ensuring that patients are fully informed.

Recent research has shown that polypharmacy resulting from inappropriate drug selection or the use of medications without a valid indication is associated with an increased incidence of DDIs. This, in turn, raises the risk of ADRs and hospitalizations, contributing to a greater economic burden for both patients and healthcare systems [8, 169].

The prevention of polypharmacy and DDIs that may cause ADRs in geriatric patients requires a systematic, multidisciplinary approach grounded in current evidence. Strategies recommended in the medical literature include:

1. The Beers criteria, together with the clinical tools STOPP/START, can help physicians identify potentially inappropriate medications and possible risks of DDIs when prescribing for geriatric patients [170, 171]. The STOPP/START criteria are particularly valuable, as they take into account physiological systems and emphasize periodic reviews of all prescribed drugs, including over-the-counter medications and supplements. These tools prioritize the assessment and the development of an individualized care plan, involving both the patient and the multidisciplinary healthcare team, in line with comprehensive medication management.

2. Implement deprescribing processes, that is, the planned and supervised withdrawal of non-essential or high-risk medications, especially in patients with multimorbidity and limited life expectancy. This process should be individualized and aligned with the patient's therapeutic goals and preferences, involving pharmacists and other members of the healthcare team [172, 173]. Therefore, it is advisable to consult algorithms, particularly for drugs that may cause tolerance and dependence, such as antipsychotics and opioid analgesics, since strategies for gradual withdrawal can vary depending on the type of medication [174].

3. Perform medication reconciliation at every care transition (admission, discharge, outpatient visit), identifying duplications, DDIs, and prescribing errors. This practice is especially important in settings such as emergency departments and primary care [171].

4. Incorporate comprehensive geriatric assessment to identify vulnerabilities and age-related changes in pharmacokinetics and pharmacodynamics, and adjust pharmacotherapy according to the patient's renal, hepatic, and cognitive function, as well as overall functional status [175].

5. Use Clinical Decision Support Systems (CDSS), evidence-based software programs that integrate patient-specific information at the point of care [176], to assist healthcare professionals in achieving diagnostic precision and optimizing the effectiveness of pharmacological treatments [170, 171]. Alongside these tools, advances in the application of artificial intelligence (AI) strategies, such as mining large volumes of complex data, allow for the prediction of DDIs and promote more efficient, accurate, and comprehensive pharmacovigilance. These developments ultimately enhance patient safety and support the rational use of medications [177, 178].

6. Promote collaboration among physicians, pharmacists, nurses, and other professionals—particularly in nursing homes and home care—to optimize pharmacotherapy and reduce risks [56, 173]. This includes training prescribers and educating patients about regulatory measures, such as black box warnings, which are prominently displayed on drug labels and highlight specific risks, including monitoring requirements or restrictions on use. Examples include common black box warnings for certain antidepressants (suicidal thoughts), opioids (addiction, overdose), and some antibiotics (tendon rupture) [179]. All of these measures are part of risk minimization programs [180], which should be considered in every prescription and at each transition of care.

7. In addition, it is essential to consider other strategies based on the principles of rational prescribing [181]. Particularly in chronic treatments involving drugs with a high potential for interaction, it is advisable to start with a low dose, proceed gradually, and discontinue therapy whenever possible. Maintaining close communication with the patient is also critical to foster health literacy strategies, which can help minimize risks in prescribing [182].

These strategies, supported by the medical literature, have been shown to reduce the incidence of adverse reactions, hospitalizations, and complications associated with polypharmacy in older adults.

ADRs can have direct economic implications due to the increased rates of hospitalization, morbidity, mortality, and associated costs [183]. They may also negatively affect family finances through potential loss of work, caregiver burden, and changes in family dynamics. In addition, ADRs place added financial stress on healthcare systems [184], especially in developing countries.

Therefore, the effective implementation of preventive strategies requires institutional commitment and the integration of review and prescribing processes into daily clinical practice [185, 186].

5. Future perspectives

Let us imagine a near-future scenario in which every older adult has a microchip containing their complete medical history, including key genetic profile data such as hepatic cytochrome subtype. At the start of a consultation, this microchip could automatically connect to software powered by AI, which would analyze the patient's clinical data and compare the evidence with the most recent advances in clinical research.

In this way, when the physician issues a prescription, the program could estimate and alert for the presence of hidden polypharmacy, the probability of DDIs and ADRs, and encourage rational polypharmacy, where deprescribing through algorithms is continually promoted.

Moreover, this system could also have the capacity to send and install an application on the patient's mobile phone, providing the treatment plan and a reminder system for prescription schedules. In parallel, the program could generate and schedule videos to educate the patient about their pharmacological treatment, necessary precautions when taking medications, guidelines for early detection and reporting of ADRs, and counseling to avoid foods or dietary supplements that could interact with the prescribed therapies.

All of the above is already possible today, but only in separate components: Electronic medical records exist, as do AI-based programs that can guide physicians in identifying inappropriate drugs or those at risk of drug interactions, as discussed earlier.

However, despite these advances, it remains difficult to integrate all these elements into a single program, since differences still exist in the formats used for medical records across institutions and specialties. This represents a major obstacle to continuity of care for the geriatric population, particularly when a patient is repeatedly hospitalized in different institutions or requires consultations with multiple specialties.

Having up-to-date clinical information available electronically—including pharmacological treatments—would foster greater effectiveness in therapy, medical care, and pharmacovigilance.

It is essential to give special consideration to drugs with multiple mechanisms of action because of the higher risk they pose for DDIs.

Therefore, promoting further research into metformin's ability to regulate the serotonergic and GABAergic systems in pancreatic β-cells, as well as in platelets, the immune system, and the CNS, represents a key challenge that would help clarify the possible mechanisms of interaction among drugs that share similar targets, enabling the prevention or explanation of ADRs. In addition, leveraging this knowledge to innovate and explore the potential of biguanides in the treatment of other diseases is essential.

Statins and SSRIs, due to their multiple mechanisms of action, may indirectly affect SS function—statins by altering extracellular 5-HT levels, and SSRIs by lowering cholesterol levels. Both mechanisms could impact the functionality of the serotonergic system. Further research on these drugs would therefore improve the understanding of SS-related DDIs.

6. Conclusions

Biguanides, statins, and SSRIs, through their polypharmacological actions, may interact directly or indirectly with the SS, which is present in various systems including the gastrointestinal tract, pancreas, platelets, and CNS.

Prescribing a drug with multiple mechanisms of action as part of polypharmacy in the geriatric population may significantly increase the risk of DDIs associated with adverse drug reactions (ADRs).

It is important to note that in hidden polypharmacy the risks of adverse effects are often underestimated, highlighting the need to strengthen individualized pharmacovigilance strategies based on effective communication between healthcare professionals and patients, fostering training for the former and education for the latter.

Therefore, before prescribing any drug with polypharmacological properties, its use should be carefully evaluated and, whenever possible, reconsidered. If prescribing is necessary, both family members and healthcare professionals must remain vigilant for the appearance of ADRs in order to ensure timely intervention and prevent serious outcomes.

Author details

Alfredo Briones-Aranda
Facultad de Medicina Humana, Universidad Autónoma de Chiapas, Mexico

*Address all correspondence to: alfredo.briones@unach.mx; alfred725@hotmail.com

References

[1] Patel N, Yeboah J. Multimorbidity in the era of increasing life expectancy and aging population. European Journal of Heart Failure. 2024;**26**(4):869-870

[2] Lauder L, Mahfoud F, Azizi M, Bhatt DL, Ewen S, Kario K, et al. Hypertension management in patients with cardiovascular comorbidities. European Heart Journal. 2023;**44**(23):2066-2077

[3] Abdelhafiz AH. Diabetic kidney disease in older people with type 2 diabetes mellitus: Improving prevention and treatment options. Drugs & Aging. 2020;**37**(8):567-584

[4] Masnoon N, Shakib S, Kalisch-Ellett L, Caughey GE. What is polypharmacy? A systematic review of definitions. BMC Geriatrics. 2017;**17**(1):230

[5] Bushardt R. Polypharmacy: Misleading, but manageable. Clinical Interventions in Aging. 2008;**3**:383-389

[6] Maher RL, Hanlon J, Hajjar ER. Clinical consequences of polypharmacy in elderly. Expert Opinion on Drug Safety. 2014;**13**(1):57-65

[7] Cho HJ, Chae J, Yoon SH, Kim DS. Factors related to polypharmacy and hyper-polypharmacy for the elderly: A nationwide cohort study using National Health Insurance data in South Korea. Clinical and Translational Science. 2023;**16**(2):193-205

[8] Woodford HJ. Polypharmacy in older patients. British Journal of Hospital Medicine (London, England). 2024;**85**(10):1-12

[9] Zhang N, Sundquist J, Sundquist K, Ji J. An increasing trend in the prevalence of polypharmacy in Sweden: A Nationwide register-based study. Frontiers in Pharmacology. 2020;**11**:326

[10] Bojuwoye AO, Suleman F, Perumal-Pillay VA. Polypharmacy and the occurrence of potential drug-drug interactions among geriatric patients at the outpatient pharmacy department of a regional hospital in Durban, South Africa. Journal of Pharmaceutical Policy and Practice. 2022;**15**(1):1

[11] Błeszyńska-Marunowska E, Wierucki Ł, Jagiełło K, Rewiuk K, Mitręga K, Kalarus Z. Prevalence and factors predisposing to potential drug-drug interactions in a polish community-dwelling geriatric population: An observational, cross-sectional study. Advances in Clinical and Experimental Medicine. 2023;**32**(3):331-339

[12] Laatikainen O, Sneck S, Bloigu R, Lahtinen M, Lauri T, Turpeinen M. Hospitalizations due to adverse drug events in the elderly-a retrospective register study. Frontiers in Pharmacology. 2016;**7**:358

[13] Shi Q, Tong Y, Zheng Y, Liu Y, Yin T. PDT-sensitized ROS-responsive dextran nanosystem for maximizing antitumor potency of multi-target drugs. International Journal of Pharmaceutics. 2023;**633**:122567

[14] Conley AC, Newhouse PA. Advances in drug discovery and development in geriatric psychiatry. Current Psychiatry Reports. 2018;**20**(2):10

[15] Morrison PD, Jauhar S, Young AH. The mechanism of action of clozapine. Journal of Psychopharmacology. 2025;**39**(4):297-300

[16] Nan X, Xie C, Yu X, Liu J. EGFR TKI as first-line treatment for patients with advanced EGFR mutation-positive non-small-cell lung cancer. Oncotarget. 2017;**8**(43):75712-75726

[17] Hamada S, Gulliford MC. Drug prescribing during the last year of life in very old people with diabetes. Age and Ageing. 2016;**46**(1):147-151

[18] Jyrkkä J, Enlund H, Lavikainen P, Sulkava R, Hartikainen S. Association of polypharmacy with nutritional status, functional ability and cognitive capacity over a three-year period in an elderly population. Pharmacoepidemiology and Drug Safety. 2011;**20**(5):514-522

[19] Tromp AM, Pluijm SMF, Smit JH, Deeg DJH, Bouter LM, Lips P. Fall-risk screening test. Journal of Clinical Epidemiology. 2001;**54**(8):837-844

[20] Heuberger RA, Caudell K. Polypharmacy and nutritional status in older adults. Drugs & Aging. 2011;**28**(4):315-323

[21] Malet-Larrea A, Goyenechea E, García-Cárdenas V, Calvo B, Arteche JM, Aranegui P, et al. The impact of a medication review with follow-up service on hospital admissions in aged polypharmacy patients. British Journal of Clinical Pharmacology. 2016;**82**(3):831-838

[22] Brick N, Daniels J, Jenkins K, Iles D, Farmer C. Joint working with hospice teams: A renal collaborative approach. EDTNA ERCA J. 2005;**31**(2):88-92

[23] Keshavarz M, Xie K, Bano D, Ehninger D. Aging - what it is and how to measure it. Mechanisms of Ageing and Development. 2023;**213**:111837

[24] Mangoni AA, Jackson SHD. Age-related changes in pharmacokinetics and pharmacodynamics: Basic principles and practical applications. British Journal of Clinical Pharmacology. 2004;**57**(1):6-14

[25] Méndez-Lucio Oscar J, Naveja J, Vite-Caritino H, Prieto-Martínez FD, Medina-Franco JL, Review. One drug for multiple targets: A computational perspective. Journal of the Mexican Chemical Society. 2016;**60**(3):168-181

[26] Aronson JK. In defence of polypharmacy. British Journal of Clinical Pharmacology. 2004;**57**(2):119-120

[27] Pitkälä KH, Suominen MH, Bell JS, Strandberg TE. Herbal medications and other dietary supplements. A clinical review for physicians caring for older people. Annals of Medicine. 2016;**48**(8):586-602

[28] Feldman M, Cryer B, McArthur KE, Huet BA, Lee E. Effects of aging and gastritis on gastric acid and pepsin secretion in humans: A prospective study. Gastroenterology. 1996;**110**(4):1043-1052

[29] Ishimura N, Owada Y, Aimi M, Oshima T, Kamada T, Inoue K, et al. No increase in gastric acid secretion in healthy Japanese over the past two decades. Journal of Gastroenterology. 2015;**50**(8):844-852

[30] Goldschmiedt M, Barnett CC, Schwarz BE, Karnes WE, Redfern JS, Feldman M. Effect of age on gastric acid secretion and serum gastrin concentrations in healthy men and women. Gastroenterology. 1991;**101**(4):977-990

[31] Russell RM. Gastric hypochlorhydria and achlorhydria in older adults. Journal of the American Medical Association. 1997;**278**(20):1659-1660

[32] Hurwitz A, Brady DA, Schaal SE, Samloff IM, Dedon J, Ruhl CE. Gastric

acidity in older adults. Journal of the American Medical Association. 1997;**278**(8):659-662

[33] Adachi M, Hinatsu Y, Kusamori K, Katsumi H, Sakane T, Nakatani M, et al. Improved dissolution and absorption of ketoconazole in the presence of organic acids as pH-modifiers. European Journal of Pharmaceutical Sciences. 2015;**76**:225-230

[34] Ahmed T, Haboubi N. Assessment and management of nutrition in older people and its importance to health. Clinical Interventions in Aging. 2010;**5**:207-216

[35] Lu H, Ayers E, Patel P, Mattoo TK. Body water percentage from childhood to old age. Kidney Research and Clinical Practice. 2023;**42**(3):340-348

[36] Mian P, Allegaert K, Spriet I, Tibboel D, Petrovic M. Paracetamol in older people: Towards evidence-based dosing? Drugs & Aging. 2018;**35**(7):603-624

[37] Klotz U, Avant GR, Hoyumpa A, Schenker S, Wilkinson GR. The effects of age and liver disease on the disposition and elimination of diazepam in adult man. The Journal of Clinical Investigation. 1975;**55**(2):347-359

[38] Björkman S, Wada DR, Berling BM, Benoni G. Prediction of the disposition of midazolam in surgical patients by a physiologically based pharmacokinetic model. Journal of Pharmaceutical Sciences. 2001;**90**(9):1226-1241

[39] Greenblatt DJ. Reduced serum albumin concentration in the elderly: A report from the Boston collaborative drug surveillance program. Journal of the American Geriatrics Society. 1979;**27**(1):20-22

[40] Jiang Y, Yang Z, Wu Q, Cao J, Qiu T. The association between albumin and C-reactive protein in older adults. Medicine. 2023;**102**(34):e34726

[41] Bowden RG, Wilson RL. Malnutrition, inflammation, and lipids in a cohort of dialysis patients. Postgraduate Medicine. 2010;**122**(3):196-202

[42] Shi S, Klotz U. Age-related changes in pharmacokinetics. Current Drug Metabolism. 2011;**12**(7):601-610

[43] Wu X, Sia JEV, Hai M, Lai X, Li H, Cui C, et al. Physiologically based pharmacokinetic model for older adults and its application in geriatric drug research. Current Drug Metabolism. 2023;**24**(3):211-222

[44] Braillon A, Jirón MI, Valla D, Calès P, Lebrec D. Effect of propranolol on hepatic blood flow in patients with cirrhosis. Clinical Pharmacology and Therapeutics. 1985;**37**(4):376-380

[45] Pirttiaho HI, Sotaniemi EA, Pelkonen RO, Pitkänen U, Anttila M, Sundqvist H. Roles of hepatic blood flow and enzyme activity in the kinetics of propranolol and sotalol. British Journal of Clinical Pharmacology. 1980;**9**(4):399-405

[46] Parker RB, Laizure SC. The effect of ethanol on oral cocaine pharmacokinetics reveals an unrecognized class of ethanol-mediated drug interactions. Drug Metabolism and Disposition. 2010;**38**(2):317-322

[47] Klotz U. Pharmacokinetics and drug metabolism in the elderly. Drug Metabolism Reviews. 2009;**41**(2):67-76

[48] Benedetti M, Whomsley R, Canning M. Drug metabolism in the paediatric population and in

the elderly. Drug Discovery Today. 2007;**12**(15-16):599-610

[49] Zhang Y, Wang Z, Wang Y, Jin W, Zhang Z, Jin L, et al. CYP3A4 and CYP3A5: The crucial roles in clinical drug metabolism and the significant implications of genetic polymorphisms. PeerJ. 2024;**12**:e18636

[50] Hernández-Lorca M, Timón IM, Ballester P, Henarejos-Escudero P, García-Muñoz AM, Victoria-Montesinos D, et al. Dietary modulation of CYP3A4 and its impact on statins and antidiabetic drugs: A narrative Review. Pharmaceuticals. 2025;**18**(9):1351

[51] Benz MB, Epstein-Lubow G, Weinstock LM, Gaudiano BA. Polypharmacy among patients with major depressive disorder and Co-occurring substance use disorders in a psychiatric hospital setting. Journal of Clinical Psychopharmacology. 2023;**43**(3):273-277

[52] Sokol KC, Knudsen JF, Li MM. Polypharmacy in older oncology patients and the need for an interdisciplinary approach to side-effect management. Journal of Clinical Pharmacy and Therapeutics. 2007;**32**(2):169-175

[53] Lennernäs H. Clinical pharmacokinetics of atorvastatin. Clinical Pharmacokinetics. 2003;**42**(13):1141-1160

[54] Taylor C, Crosby I, Yip V, Maguire P, Pirmohamed M, Turner RM. A Review of the important role of CYP2D6 in pharmacogenomics. Genes (Basel). 2020;**11**(11):1295

[55] Corsonello A, Pedone C, Incalzi R. Age-related pharmacokinetic and Pharmacodynamic changes and related risk of adverse drug reactions. Current Medicinal Chemistry. 2010;**17**(6):571-584

[56] Damluji AA, Forman DE, Wang TY, Chikwe J, Kunadian V, Rich MW, et al. Management of Acute Coronary Syndrome in the older adult population: A scientific statement from the American Heart Association. Circulation. 2023;**147**(3):e32-e62

[57] Ngcobo NN. Influence of ageing on the pharmacodynamics and pharmacokinetics of chronically administered medicines in geriatric patients: A Review. Clinical Pharmacokinetics. 2025;**64**(3):463

[58] Mühlberg W, Platt D. Age-dependent changes of the kidneys: Pharmacological implications. Gerontology. 1999;**45**(5): 243-253

[59] Turnheim K. When drug therapy gets old: Pharmacokinetics and pharmacodynamics in the elderly. Experimental Gerontology. 2003;**38**(8):843-853

[60] Turnheim K. Drug therapy in the elderly. Experimental Gerontology. 2004;**39**(11-12):1731-1738

[61] Dreischulte T, Morales DR, Bell S, Guthrie B. Combined use of nonsteroidal anti-inflammatory drugs with diuretics and/or renin–angiotensin system inhibitors in the community increases the risk of acute kidney injury. Kidney International. 2015;**88**(2):396-403

[62] Gigante A, Proietti M, Petrillo E, Mannucci PM, Nobili A, Muscaritoli M. Renal function, cardiovascular diseases, appropriateness of drug prescription and outcomes in hospitalized older patients. Drugs & Aging. 2021;**38**(12):1097-1105

[63] Mörike K, Schwab M, Klotz U. Use of aminoglycosides in elderly patients. Drugs & Aging. 1997;**10**(4):259-277

[64] Tobita S, Sogawa R, Murakawa T, Kimura S, Tasaki M, Sakamoto Y, et al. The importance of monitoring renal function and concomitant medication to avoid toxicity in patients taking lithium. International Clinical Psychopharmacology. 2021;**36**(1):34-37

[65] Corsonello A, Onder G, Bustacchini S, Provinciali M, Garasto S, Gareri P, et al. Estimating renal function to reduce the risk of adverse drug reactions. Drug Safety. 2012;**35**(S1): 47-54

[66] Graham GG, Punt J, Arora M, Day RO, Doogue MP, Duong JK, et al. Clinical pharmacokinetics of metformin. Clinical Pharmacokinetics. 2011;**50**(2):81-98

[67] Markowicz-Piasecka M, Huttunen KM, Mateusiak L, Mikiciuk-Olasik E, Sikora J. Is metformin a perfect drug? Updates in pharmacokinetics and pharmacodynamics. Current Pharmaceutical Design. 2017;**23**(17):2532-2550

[68] Wróbel MP, Marek B, Kajdaniuk D, Rokicka D, Szymborska-Kajanek A, Strojek K. Metformin - a new old drug. Endokrynologia Polska. 2017;**68**(4):482-496

[69] McCreight LJ, Bailey CJ, Pearson ER. Metformin and the gastrointestinal tract. Diabetologia. 2016;**59**(3):426-435

[70] Tarasova L, Kalnina I, Geldnere K, Bumbure A, Ritenberga R, Nikitina-Zake L, et al. Association of genetic variation in the organic cation transporters OCT1, OCT2 and multidrug and toxin extrusion 1 transporter protein genes with the gastrointestinal side effects and lower BMI in metformin-treated type 2 diabetes patients. Pharmacogenetics and Genomics. 2012;**22**(9):659-666

[71] Kim A, Chung I, Yoon SH, Yu KS, Lim KS, Cho JY, et al. Effects of proton pump inhibitors on metformin pharmacokinetics and pharmacodynamics. Drug Metabolism and Disposition. 2014;**42**(7):1174-1179

[72] Nies AT, Hofmann U, Resch C, Schaeffeler E, Rius M, Schwab M. Proton pump inhibitors inhibit metformin uptake by organic cation transporters (OCTs). PLoS One. 2011;**6**(7):e22163

[73] Domagała-Rodacka R, Cibor D, Szczeklik K, Rodacki T, Mach T, Owczarek D. Gastrointestinal tract as a side-effect target of medications. Przegląd Lekarski. 2016;**73**(9):652-658

[74] Wu T, Xie C, Wu H, Jones KL, Horowitz M, Rayner CK. Metformin reduces the rate of small intestinal glucose absorption in type 2 diabetes. Diabetes, Obesity & Metabolism. 2017;**19**(2):290-293

[75] Bouchoucha M, Uzzan B, Cohen R. Metformin and digestive disorders. Diabetes & Metabolism. 2011;**37**(2):90-96

[76] Caspary WF, Zavada I, Reimold W, Deuticke U, Emrich D, Willms B. Alteration of bile acid metabolism and vitamin-B12-absorption in diabetics on biguanides. Diabetologia. 1977;**13**(3):187-193

[77] Hermans MP, Ahn SA, Rousseau MF. What is the phenotype of patients with gastrointestinal intolerance to metformin? Diabetes & Metabolism. 2013;**39**(4):322-329

[78] Chaudhary M, Midha NK, Sukhadiya P, Kumar D, Garg MK. Metformin-induced chronic diarrhea misdiagnosed as irritable bowel syndrome for years. Cureus. 2024;**16**(3):e56828

[79] Bettge K, Kahle M, Abd El Aziz MS, Meier JJ, Nauck MA. Occurrence of nausea, vomiting and diarrhoea reported as adverse events in clinical trials studying glucagon-like peptide-1 receptor agonists: A systematic analysis of published clinical trials. Diabetes, Obesity & Metabolism. 2017;**19**(3):336-347

[80] Cubeddu LX, Bönisch H, Göthert M, Molderings G, Racké K, Ramadori G, et al. Effects of metformin on intestinal 5-hydroxytryptamine (5-HT) release and on 5-HT3 receptors. Naunyn-Schmiedeberg's Archives of Pharmacology. 2000;**361**(1):85-91

[81] Hoffmann IS, Roa M, Torrico F, Cubeddu LX. Ondansetron and metformin-induced gastrointestinal side effects. American Journal of Therapeutics. 2003;**10**(6):447-451

[82] Pecikoza U, Lasica A, Nastić K, Dinić M, Jasnić N, Micov A, et al. Metformin reduces inflammatory nociception in mice through a serotonin-dependent mechanism. European Journal of Pharmacology. 2025;**991**:177324

[83] Fujitsuka N, Asakawa A, Hayashi M, Sameshima M, Amitani H, Kojima S, et al. Selective serotonin reuptake inhibitors modify physiological gastrointestinal motor activities via 5-HT2c receptor and acyl ghrelin. Biological Psychiatry. 2009;**65**(9):748-759

[84] Madiraju AK, Erion DM, Rahimi Y, Zhang XM, Braddock DT, Albright RA, et al. Metformin suppresses gluconeogenesis by inhibiting mitochondrial glycerophosphate dehydrogenase. Nature. 2014;**510**(7506):542-546

[85] Franzetti I, Paolo D, Marco G, Emanuela M, Elisabetta Z, Renato U. Possible synergistic effect of metformin and enalapril on the development of hyperkaliemic lactic acidosis. Diabetes Research and Clinical Practice. 1997;**38**(3):173-176

[86] Palmer BF, Clegg DJ. Electrolyte and Acid–Base disturbances in patients with diabetes mellitus. New England Journal of Medicine. 2015;**373**(6):548-559

[87] Gudmundsdottir H, Aksnes H, Heldal K, Krogh A, Froyshov S, Rudberg N, et al. Metformin and antihypertensive therapy with drugs blocking the renin angiotensin system, a cause of concern? Clinical Nephrology. 2006;**66**(5):380-385

[88] DeFronzo R, Fleming GA, Chen K, Bicsak TA. Metformin-associated lactic acidosis: Current perspectives on causes and risk. Metabolism. 2016;**65**(2):20-29

[89] Di Mauro S, Filippello A, Scamporrino A, Purrello F, Piro S, Malaguarnera R. Metformin: When should we fear lactic acidosis? International Journal of Molecular Sciences. 2022;**23**(15):8320

[90] Galicia-Garcia U, Benito-Vicente A, Jebari S, Larrea-Sebal A, Siddiqi H, Uribe KB, et al. Pathophysiology of type 2 diabetes mellitus. International Journal of Molecular Sciences. 2020;**21**(17):6275

[91] Bjornstad P, Choi YJ, Platnick C, Gross S, Narongkiatikhun P, Melena I, et al. Insulin secretion, sensitivity, and kidney function in Young individuals with type 2 diabetes. Diabetes Care. 2024;**47**(3):409-417

[92] Lundquist I, Mohammed Al-Amily I, Meidute Abaraviciene S, Salehi A. Metformin ameliorates dysfunctional traits of Glibenclamide- and glucose-induced insulin secretion by suppression of imposed Overactivity of the islet nitric

oxide synthase-NO system. PLoS One. 2016;**11**(11):e0165668

[93] American Diabetes Association Professional Practice Committee. 9. Pharmacologic approaches to glycemic treatment: Standards of Care in Diabetes-2025. Diabetes Care. 2025;**48**(1 Suppl 1):S181-S206

[94] Zhang Q, Zhu Y, Zhou W, Gao L, Yuan L, Han X. Serotonin receptor 2C and insulin secretion. PLoS One. 2013;**8**(1):e54250

[95] Om A, Baquero A, Raja R, Kim P, Bannett AD. The prognostic significance of the presence of monocytes in glomeruli of renal transplant allografts. Transplantation Proceedings. 1987;**19**(1 Pt 2):1618-1622

[96] Golubic R, Hussein Ismail M, Josipovic M, Kennet J, Galderisi A, Evans ML. Sumatriptan, a serotonin 5HT1B receptor agonist, acutely reduces insulin secretion and sensitivity and glucose effectiveness in overweight humans: A double-blinded placebo-controlled cross-over trial. Diabetes, Obesity & Metabolism. 2023;**25**(10):3059-3063

[97] Ieni JR, Meyerson LR. The 5-HT1A receptor probe [3H]8-OH-DPAT labels the 5-HT transporter in human platelets. Life Sciences. 1988;**42**(3):311-320

[98] Berry CN, Lorrain J, Lochot S, Delahaye M, Lalé A, Savi P, et al. Antiplatelet and antithrombotic activity of SL65.0472, a mixed 5-HT1B/5-HT2A receptor antagonist. Thrombosis and Haemostasis. 2001;**85**(3):521-528

[99] Moerland M, Kemme M, Dijkmans A, Bergougnan L, Burggraaf J. Modulation of vasoactivity and platelet aggregation by selective 5-HT receptor antagonism in humans. Journal of Cardiovascular Pharmacology. 2011;**58**(6):575-580

[100] Braun M, Ramracheya R, Bengtsson M, Clark A, Walker JN, Johnson PR, et al. γ-Aminobutyric acid (GABA) is an autocrine excitatory transmitter in human pancreatic β-cells. Diabetes. 2010;**59**(7):1694-1701

[101] Untereiner A, Xu J, Bhattacharjee A, Cabrera O, Hu C, Dai FF, et al. γ-Aminobutyric acid stimulates β-cell proliferation through the mTORC1/p70S6K pathway, an effect amplified by Ly49, a novel γ-aminobutyric acid type a receptor positive allosteric modulator. Diabetes, Obesity & Metabolism. 2020;**22**(11):2021-2031

[102] Al-Kuraishy HM, Hussian NR, Al-Naimi MS, Al-Gareeb AI, Al-Mamorri F, Al-Buhadily AK. The potential role of pancreatic γ-aminobutyric acid (GABA) in diabetes mellitus: A critical reappraisal. International Journal of Preventive Medicine. 2021;**12**:19

[103] Fan J, Li D, Chen HS, Huang JG, Xu JF, Zhu WW, et al. Metformin produces anxiolytic-like effects in rats by facilitating GABAA receptor trafficking to membrane. British Journal of Pharmacology. 2019;**176**(2):297-316

[104] Meneses A. Stimulation of 5-HT1A, 5-HT1B, 5-HT2A/2C, 5-HT3 and 5-HT4 receptors or 5-HT uptake inhibition: Short- and long-term memory. Behavioural Brain Research. 2007;**184**(1):81-90

[105] Ruf B, Bhagwagar Z. The 5-HT1B receptor: A novel target for the pathophysiology of depression (supplementary tables). Current Drug Targets. 2009;**10**(11):1118-1138

[106] Yu XD, Zhu Y, Sun QX, Deng F, Wan J, Zheng D, et al. Distinct serotonergic pathways to the amygdala underlie separate behavioral features of anxiety. Nature Neuroscience. 2022;**25**(12):1651-1663

[107] Luo C, Yu XM, Zeng MQ, Duan CZ, Xu SY, Zhu CY, et al. Breaking the diabetes-depression cycle: Exploring shared mechanisms, neuroinflammation, and emerging interventions for metabolic-mood comorbidities. World Journal of Diabetes. 2025;**16**(7):107406

[108] Koch CG. Statin therapy. Current Pharmaceutical Design. 2012;**18**(38):6284-6290

[109] Cilla DD, Gibson DM, Whitfield LR, Sedman AJ. Pharmacodynamic effects and pharmacokinetics of atorvastatin after administration to normocholesterolemic subjects in the morning and evening. Journal of Clinical Pharmacology. 1996;**36**(7):604-609

[110] Stillemans G, Paquot A, Muccioli GG, Hoste E, Panin N, Åsberg A, et al. Atorvastatin population pharmacokinetics in a real-life setting: Influence of genetic polymorphisms and association with clinical response. Clinical and Translational Science. 2022;**15**(3):667-679

[111] Ray KK, Cannon CP, McCabe CH, Cairns R, Tonkin AM, Sacks FM, et al. Early and late benefits of high-dose atorvastatin in patients with acute coronary syndromes: Results from the PROVE IT-TIMI 22 trial. Journal of the American College of Cardiology. 2005;**46**(8):1405-1410

[112] Stone NJ, Robinson JG, Lichtenstein AH, Bairey Merz CN, Blum CB, Eckel RH, et al. ACC/AHA guideline on the treatment of blood cholesterol to reduce atherosclerotic cardiovascular risk in adults: A report of the American College of Cardiology/American Heart Association task force on practice guidelines. Journal of the American College of Cardiology 2014. 2013;**63**(25 Pt B):2889-2934

[113] Shin J, Pauly DF, Pacanowski MA, Langaee T, Frye RF, Johnson JA. Effect of cytochrome P450 3A5 genotype on atorvastatin pharmacokinetics and its interaction with clarithromycin. Pharmacotherapy. 2011;**31**(10):942-950

[114] Hougaard Christensen MM, Bruun Haastrup M, Øhlenschlaeger T, Esbech P, Arnspang Pedersen S, Bach Dunvald AC, et al. Interaction potential between clarithromycin and individual statins-a systematic review. Basic & Clinical Pharmacology & Toxicology. 2020;**126**(4):307-317

[115] Amundsen R, Christensen H, Zabihyan B, Asberg A. Cyclosporine a, but not tacrolimus, shows relevant inhibition of organic anion-transporting protein 1B1-mediated transport of atorvastatin. Drug Metabolism and Disposition. 2010;**38**(9):1499-1504

[116] He YJ, Zhang W, Chen Y, Guo D, Tu JH, Xu LY, et al. Rifampicin alters atorvastatin plasma concentration on the basis of SLCO1B1 521T>C polymorphism. Clinica Chimica Acta. 2009;**405**(1-2):49-52

[117] Suthutvoravut S, Chaturachinda K. Risk of low birthweight at Ramathibodi hospital. Journal of the Medical Association of Thailand. 1988;**71**(Suppl 2):6-11

[118] Alsheikh-Ali AA, Karas RH. Safety of lovastatin/extended release niacin compared with lovastatin alone, atorvastatin alone, pravastatin alone, and simvastatin alone (from the United

States Food and Drug Administration adverse event reporting system). The American Journal of Cardiology. 2007;**99**(3):379-381

[119] Averbukh LD, Turshudzhyan A, Wu DC, Wu GY. Statin-induced liver injury patterns: A clinical Review. Journal of Clinical and Translational Hepatology. 2022;**10**(3):543-552

[120] Huang YS, Tseng SY, Chen WW, Chang TT, Peng CY, Lo GH, et al. Clinical characteristics and outcomes of drug-induced liver injury in Taiwan: With emphasis on the impact of chronic hepatitis B infection. Journal of the Chinese Medical Association. 2022;**85**(3):286-294

[121] Park S, Ishino R. Liver injury associated with antidepressants. Current Drug Safety. 2013;**8**(3):207-223

[122] Chang CY, Schiano TD. Review article: Drug hepatotoxicity. Alimentary Pharmacology & Therapeutics. 2007;**25**(10):1135-1151

[123] Sugawara T, Nomura E, Hoshi N. Cholesterol sulphate affects production of steroid hormones by reducing steroidogenic acute regulatory protein level in adrenocortical cells. The Journal of Endocrinology. 2007;**195**(3):451-458

[124] Schade DS, Shey L, Eaton RP. Cholesterol Review: A metabolically important molecule. Endocrine Practice. 2020;**26**(12):1514-1523

[125] Newman CB, Blaha MJ, Boord JB, Cariou B, Chait A, Fein HG, et al. Lipid Management in Patients with endocrine disorders: An Endocrine Society clinical practice guideline. The Journal of Clinical Endocrinology and Metabolism. 2020;**105**(12):3613-3682

[126] Oluleye OW, Kronmal RA, Folsom AR, Vaidya DM, Ouyang P, Duprez DA, et al. Association between statin use and sex hormone in the multi-ethnic study of atherosclerosis cohort. The Journal of Clinical Endocrinology and Metabolism. 2019;**104**(10):4600-4606

[127] Stamerra CA, Di Giosia P, Ferri C, Giorgini P, Reiner Z, Johnston TP, et al. Statin therapy and sex hormones. European Journal of Pharmacology. 2021;**890**:173745

[128] Anelli V, Armeni E, Paschou SA, Lambrinoudaki I. Statin use and incident type 2 diabetes mellitus in women after menopause. Maturitas. 2024;**181**:107914

[129] Hsia J, Klouj A, Prasad A, Burt J, Adams-Campbell LL, Howard BV. Progression of coronary calcification in healthy postmenopausal women. BMC Cardiovascular Disorders. 2004;**4**:21

[130] Peck A, Chaikittisilpa S, Mirzaei R, Wang J, Mack WJ, Hodis HN, et al. Effect of statins on estrogen and androgen levels in postmenopausal women treated with estradiol. Climacteric. 2011;**14**(1):49-53

[131] Krysiak R, Gilowski W, Szkrobka W, Okopien B. The effect of atorvastatin on Cardiometabolic risk factors in Bromocriptine-treated premenopausal women with isolated hypercholesterolemia. Cardiovascular Therapeutics. 2015;**33**(5):282-287

[132] Shrivastava S, Pucadyil TJ, Paila YD, Ganguly S, Chattopadhyay A. Chronic cholesterol depletion using statin impairs the function and dynamics of human serotonin 1A receptors. Biochemistry. 2010;**49**(26):5426-5435

[133] You H, Lu W, Zhao S, Hu Z, Zhang J. The relationship between statins and depression: A review of the literature. Expert Opinion on Pharmacotherapy. 2013;**14**(11):1467-1476

[134] Deveau CM, Rodriguez E, Schroering A, Yamamoto BK. Serotonin transporter regulation by cholesterol-independent lipid signaling. Biochemical Pharmacology. 2021;**183**:114349

[135] Stuart SA, Robertson JD, Marrion NV, Robinson ESJ. Chronic pravastatin but not atorvastatin treatment impairs cognitive function in two rodent models of learning and memory. PLoS One. 2013;**8**(9):e75467

[136] Baytan SH, Alkanat M, Okuyan M, Ekinci M, Gedikli E, Ozeren M, et al. Simvastatin impairs spatial memory in rats at a specific dose level. The Tohoku Journal of Experimental Medicine. 2008;**214**(4):341-349

[137] Maggo S, Ashton JC. Effects of HMG-CoA reductase inhibitors on learning and memory in the Guinea pig. European Journal of Pharmacology. 2014;**723**:294-304

[138] Pfrieger FW. Cholesterol homeostasis and function in neurons of the central nervous system. Cellular and Molecular Life Sciences. 2003;**60**(6):1158-1171

[139] Schultz BG, Patten DK, Berlau DJ. The role of statins in both cognitive impairment and protection against dementia: A tale of two mechanisms. Translational Neurodegeneration. 2018;7:5

[140] Gutierrez MG, Malmstadt N. Human serotonin receptor 5-HT(1A) preferentially segregates to the liquid disordered phase in synthetic lipid bilayers. Journal of the American Chemical Society. 2014;**136**(39):13530-13533

[141] Sjögren B, Hamblin MW, Svenningsson P. Cholesterol depletion reduces serotonin binding and signaling via human 5-HT(7(a)) receptors. European Journal of Pharmacology. 2006;**552**(1-3):1-10

[142] Zhang YY, Fan YC, Wang M, Wang D, Li XH. Atorvastatin attenuates the production of IL-1β, IL-6, and TNF-α in the hippocampus of an amyloid β1-42-induced rat model of Alzheimer's disease. Clinical Interventions in Aging. 2013;**8**:103-110

[143] Clarke WP, Maayani S. Estrogen effects on 5-HT1A receptors in hippocampal membranes from ovariectomized rats: Functional and binding studies. Brain Research. 1990;**518**(1-2):287-291

[144] Zhou Z, Ryan J, Ernst ME, Zoungas S, Tonkin AM, Woods RL, et al. Effect of statin therapy on cognitive decline and incident dementia in older adults. Journal of the American College of Cardiology. 2021;**77**(25):3145-3156

[145] McGuinness B, Craig D, Bullock R, Passmore P. Statins for the prevention of dementia. Cochrane Database of Systematic Reviews. 2016;**2016**(1):CD003160

[146] Edinoff AN, Raveendran K, Colon MA, Thomas BH, Trettin KA, Hunt GW, et al. Selective serotonin reuptake inhibitors and associated bleeding risks: A narrative and clinical Review. Health. Psychological Research. 2022;**10**(4):39580

[147] Knorr U, Madsen JM, Kessing LV. The effect of selective serotonin reuptake inhibitors in healthy subjects revisited: A systematic review of the literature. Experimental and Clinical Psychopharmacology. 2019;**27**(5):413-432

[148] Tan JY, Levin GM. Citalopram in the treatment of depression and

other potential uses in psychiatry. Pharmacotherapy: The Journal of Human Pharmacology and Drug Therapy. 1999;**19**(6):675-689

[149] Barakat A, Hamdy MM, Elbadr MM. Uses of fluoxetine in nociceptive pain management: A literature overview. European Journal of Pharmacology. 2018;**829**:12-25

[150] Moisset X. Neuropathic pain: Evidence based recommendations. Presse Médicale. 2024;**53**(2):104232

[151] Kraus C, Castrén E, Kasper S, Lanzenberger R. Serotonin and neuroplasticity – Links between molecular, functional and structural pathophysiology in depression. Neuroscience and Biobehavioral Reviews. 2017;**77**:317-326

[152] Vahid-Ansari F, Albert PR. Rewiring of the serotonin system in major depression. Frontiers in Psychiatry. 2021:12

[153] Bennett A, Maxwell R. Synapse regression in depression: The role of 5-HT receptors in modulating NMDA receptor function and synaptic plasticity. Australian & New Zealand Journal of Psychiatry. 2010;**44**(4):301-308

[154] Cremers TIFH, Giorgetti M, Bosker FJ, Hogg S, Arnt J, Mørk A, et al. Inactivation of 5-HT2C receptors potentiates consequences of serotonin reuptake blockade. Neuropsychopharmacology. 2004;**29**(10):1782-1789

[155] Sotty F, Folgering JHA, Brennum LT, Hogg S, Mørk A, Hertel P, et al. Relevance of dorsal raphe nucleus firing in serotonin 5-HT2C receptor blockade-induced augmentation of SSRIs effects. Neuropharmacology. 2009;**57**(1):18-24

[156] Demireva EY, Suri D, Morelli E, Mahadevia D, Chuhma N, Teixeira CM, et al. 5-HT2C receptor blockade reverses SSRI-associated basal ganglia dysfunction and potentiates therapeutic efficacy. Molecular Psychiatry. 2020;**25**(12):3304-3321

[157] Pacher P, Kecskemeti V. Cardiovascular side effects of new antidepressants and antipsychotics: New drugs, old concerns? Current Pharmaceutical Design. 2004;**10**(20):2463-2475

[158] Leach MJ, Pratt NL, Roughead EE. Risk of hip fracture in older people using selective serotonin reuptake inhibitors and other psychoactive medicines concurrently: A matched case–control study in Australia. Drugs Real World Outcomes. 2017;**4**(2):87-96

[159] Fryer JD, Lukas RJ. Antidepressants noncompetitively inhibit nicotinic acetylcholine receptor function. Journal of Neurochemistry. 1999;**72**(3):1117-1124

[160] Jiang HY, Chen HZ, Hu XJ, Yu ZH, Yang W, Deng M, et al. Use of selective serotonin reuptake inhibitors and risk of upper gastrointestinal bleeding: A systematic review and meta-analysis. Clinical Gastroenterology and Hepatology. 2015;**13**(1):42-50.e3

[161] Strubel T, Birkhofer A, Mössmer G, Förstl H. SSRI - treatment and bleeding. What risks do we take? Der Nervenarzt. 2010;**81**(5):549-555

[162] Andrade C, Sharma E. Serotonin reuptake inhibitors and risk of abnormal bleeding. The Psychiatric Clinics of North America. 2016;**39**(3):413-426

[163] Gregory JM, Rosenblat JD, McIntyre RS. Deconstructing diabetes and depression: Clinical context, treatment strategies, and new

directions. Focus (American Psychiatric Publishing). 2016;**14**(2):184-193

[164] Matsuura T, Tawfik AG, Ben-Umeh KC, Hansten PD, Malone DC. Evaluation of hyponatremia among older adults exposed to selective serotonin reuptake inhibitors and thiazide diuretics. Pharmacotherapy. 2025;**45**(3):169-176

[165] Humbert X, Fedrizzi S, Chrétien B, Sassier M, Bagheri H, Combret S, et al. Hypertension induced by serotonin reuptake inhibitors: Analysis of two pharmacovigilance databases. Fundamental & Clinical Pharmacology. 2019;**33**(3):296-302

[166] van Haelst IMM, van Klei WA, Doodeman HJ, Kalkman CJ, Egberts TCG. Selective serotonin reuptake inhibitors and intraoperative blood pressure. American Journal of Hypertension. 2012;**25**(2):223-228

[167] Beach SR, Kostis WJ, Celano CM, Januzzi JL, Ruskin JN, Noseworthy PA, et al. Meta-analysis of selective serotonin reuptake inhibitor-associated QTc prolongation. The Journal of Clinical Psychiatry. 2014;**75**(5):e441-e449

[168] Crépeau-Gendron G, Brown HK, Shorey C, Madan R, Szabuniewicz C, Koh S, et al. Association between citalopram, escitalopram and QTc prolongation in a real-world geriatric setting. Journal of Affective Disorders. 2019;**250**:341-345

[169] Al-Maqbali JS, Al-Zakwani I. Inappropriate polypharmacy and the need for comprehensive medication management service. Sultan Qaboos University Medical Journal. 2024;**24**(2):149-151

[170] Kurczewska-Michalak M, Lewek P, Jankowska-Polańska B, Giardini A, Granata N, Maffoni M, et al. Polypharmacy Management in the Older Adults: A scoping Review of available interventions. Frontiers in Pharmacology. 2021;**12**:734045

[171] Petrovic M, O'Mahony D, Cherubini A. Inappropriate prescribing: Hazards and solutions. Age and Ageing. 2022;**51**(2):afab269

[172] Scott IA, Hilmer SN, Reeve E, Potter K, Le Couteur D, Rigby D, et al. Reducing inappropriate polypharmacy. JAMA. Internal Medicine. 2015;**175**(5):827

[173] Hoel RW, Giddings Connolly RM, Takahashi PY. Polypharmacy Management in Older Patients. Mayo Clinic Proceedings. 2021;**96**(1):242-256

[174] Horowitz MA, Jauhar S, Natesan S, Murray RM, Taylor D. A method for tapering antipsychotic treatment that may minimize the risk of relapse. Schizophrenia Bulletin. 2021;**47**(4):1116-1129

[175] Kratz T, Diefenbacher A. Psychopharmacological treatment in older people: Avoiding drug interactions and polypharmacy. Deutsches Ärzteblatt International. 2019;**116**(29-30):508-518

[176] Elhaddad M, Hamam S. AI-driven clinical decision support systems: An ongoing pursuit of potential. Cureus. 2024;**16**(4):e57728

[177] Ecochard R. Effects of x-irradiation on the meiosis of Vicia faba. Mutation Research. 1966;**3**(4):314-326

[178] Shamim MA, Shamim MA, Arora P, Dwivedi P. Artificial intelligence and big data for pharmacovigilance and patient safety. Journal of Medicine, Surgery, and Public Health. 2024;**3**:100139

[179] Murphy S, Roberts R. “Black box” 101: How the Food and Drug Administration evaluates, communicates, and manages drug benefit/risk. Journal of Allergy and Clinical Immunology. 2006;**117**(1):34-39

[180] Mouchantaf R, Auth D, Moride Y, Raine J, Han SY, Smith MY. Risk management for the 21st century: Current status and future needs. Drug Safety. 2021;**44**(4):409-419

[181] Maxwell SR. Rational prescribing: The principles of drug selection. Clinical Medicine. 2016;**16**(5):459-464

[182] Hitchings AW. Monitoring drug therapy. Medicine. 2012;**40**(7):376-381

[183] Putri RA, Ikawati Z, Rahmawati F, Yasin NM. An awareness of pharmacovigilance among healthcare professionals due to an underreporting of adverse drug reactions issue: A systematic Review of the current state, obstacles, and strategy. Current Drug Safety. 2024;**19**(3):317-331

[184] Kwak MJ, Chang M, Chiadika S, Aguilar D, Avritscher E, Deshmukh A, et al. Healthcare expenditure associated with polypharmacy in older adults with cardiovascular diseases. The American Journal of Cardiology. 2022;**169**:156-158

[185] Nguyen KH, Tolia V, Hart LA. Polypharmacy in the emergency department. Clinics in Geriatric Medicine. 2022;**38**(4):727-732

[186] Ceccaroli B, Lohne O. Solar grade silicon feedstock. In: Luque A, Hegedus S, editors. Handbook of Photovoltaic Science and Engineering. 2nd ed. Chichester: Wiley; 2011. pp. 169-217. DOI: 10.1002/978047974704.ch5

Chapter 2

The Burden of Inappropriate Polypharmacy: Approaches to Improve Medication Safety

Farid A. Badria and Abdullah A. Elgazar

Abstract

Polypharmacy, defined as the concurrent use of multiple medications, has become an increasingly common feature of modern healthcare, particularly among aging populations with complex multimorbidity. While the use of multiple drugs may be clinically justified in many circumstances, the growing prevalence of medication regimens that expose patients to unnecessary risk has raised significant clinical, economic, and regulatory concerns. Adverse drug events, prescribing cascades, drug–drug interactions, and the underrecognized contribution of herb-drug interactions collectively underscore the challenges associated with contemporary pharmacotherapy. This chapter situates polypharmacy within the broader context of healthcare system pressures and evolving therapeutic paradigms, highlighting the conditions under which medication use transitions from rational complexity to avoidable harm. Established clinical practices, including pharmacotherapy vigilance, interprofessional medication review, and deprescribing frameworks, are discussed alongside emerging pharmaceutical strategies designed to streamline treatment regimens. In parallel, advances in artificial intelligence-supported clinical decision systems are considered for their potential to enhance the individualized risk assessment and support safer medication management. By integrating clinical stewardship with pharmaceutical and technological innovation, the chapter provides a cohesive perspective on addressing medication-related complexity in chronic disease management, with particular attention to minimizing preventable harm while preserving the therapeutic efficacy.

Keywords: polypharmacy, multimorbidity, deprescribing, drug–drug interactions, herb–drug interactions, adverse drug events, polypill, multi-target drug design, artificial intelligence in healthcare, medication review, patient-centered care, chronic disease management

1. Introduction

The term polypharmacy has evolved significantly from a simple quantitative measure to a more nuanced clinical concept. Historically—and still commonly in research—it is defined as the regular use of five or more medications. However, this threshold is arbitrary, with studies using varying cut-points ranging from two to as high as 11 drugs, while terms like excessive polypharmacy are often applied to the use of 10 or more medications. This lack of a standardized numerical definition has led to substantial heterogeneity in the literature, making it difficult to compare the prevalence rates and intervention outcomes across studies [1].

Recognizing these limitations, a more clinically relevant framework has emerged, guided by the World Health Organization's (WHO) broader definition of polypharmacy as "the administration of many drugs at the same time or the administration of an excessive number of drugs." This definition introduces a crucial qualitative distinction between two key types of polypharmacy. Appropriate polypharmacy refers to the evidence-based and clinically justified use of multiple medications to manage complex or multiple health conditions, where therapeutic benefits outweigh the potential risks. In such cases, each medication has a clear indication, the regimen is regularly reviewed, and the treatment is optimized to achieve the defined clinical outcomes [2]. Problematic or inappropriate polypharmacy, on the other hand, occurs when the use of multiple medications becomes potentially harmful. This may involve prescribing drugs without a clear indication, using medications where risks (such as side effects or interactions) outweigh benefits, or employing combinations that create clinical or practical challenges for the patient. It may also include potentially inappropriate medications (PIMs)—drugs with an unfavorable risk–benefit ratio in specific populations, such as older adults, as identified by criteria like the Beers List.

In contrast, problematic or inappropriate polypharmacy occurs when the use of multiple medications becomes hazardous. This may involve prescribing drugs without a clear clinical indication, using medications where risks (such as side effects or interactions) outweigh benefits, or employing drug combinations that pose harm. It can also include overly complex regimens that become unmanageable or distressing for patients. Additionally, problematic polypharmacy may involve (PIMs)—drugs with an unfavorable risk–benefit balance in older adults, as identified by tools like the Beers Criteria.

When interpreting population-level statistics in this chapter, it is important to note that most prevalence data refer to polypharmacy in the quantitative sense (e.g., ≥5 drugs), not necessarily inappropriate polypharmacy. The figures thus identify populations at higher risk of inappropriate use, adverse drug events, and non-adherence—but do not imply that all cases are harmful. Indeed, polypharmacy can be clinically appropriate and necessary for patients with multimorbidity, provided that medication regimens are continuously reviewed and optimized.

The prevalence of polypharmacy, as quantitatively defined, is a growing global phenomenon driven largely by aging populations and the increasing burden of chronic disease. While estimates vary widely—from 10 to 90%, depending on definitions and populations—clear trends exist. In the United States, the prevalence of polypharmacy (≥5 drugs) more than doubled over two decades, from 8.2% in 1999–2000 to 17.1% in 2017–2018. Among adults aged ≥65 years, the rate increased from 22.4 to 45.1% during the same period. Similar patterns are observed globally: In Canada, 30.9% of adults aged 60–79 take five or more prescription medications—nearly triple the rate in those aged 40–59. European data reflect comparable trends, with a Polish national cohort reporting polypharmacy prevalence of 43.1% in adults aged 65+ and 56.0% among those aged 80 and above [3].

Certain populations experience an even greater burden. Residents of long-term care facilities—often frail and medically complex—show rates as high as 91% for the use of ≥5 medications daily. Similarly, patients with chronic conditions such as cardiovascular disease (61.7%) and diabetes (57.7%) are disproportionately affected. Socioeconomic factors also influence prevalence, with individuals in deprived areas exhibiting higher rates of polypharmacy at younger ages due to earlier onset and clustering of chronic diseases. Another high-risk group includes patients with chronic mental health disorders, who are frequently prescribed multiple psychotropic medications associated with the substantial adverse effect profiles (**Table 1**) [4, 5].

It is important to recognize that while the clinical distinction between appropriate and inappropriate polypharmacy is fundamental, much of the large-scale epidemiological and economic research referenced in this chapter employs a purely quantitative definition (e.g., the concurrent use of ≥5 medications). In such studies, this numerical threshold serves as a pragmatic proxy for identifying populations at elevated risk. Accordingly, the reported "burdens" of polypharmacy—such as increased healthcare costs, adverse drug events, and medication non-adherence—should be interpreted as outcomes that occur disproportionately within this quantitatively defined group, where inappropriate prescribing practices are more likely to occur.

Against this background, this chapter explores polypharmacy as a defining feature of contemporary pharmacotherapy while focusing particular attention on the circumstances under which medication complexity transitions from necessary clinical management to avoidable risk. Rather than treating polypharmacy as inherently undesirable, the discussion centers on identifying and addressing forms of medication use that lack clear clinical justification, compromise patient safety, or undermine the therapeutic goals. By synthesizing epidemiological evidence, clinical stewardship approaches, and emerging pharmaceutical and digital innovations, the chapter aims to provide a cohesive perspective on how medication-related harm can be minimized without compromising effective treatment of multimorbidity. In doing so, it situates

Population*	Prevalence of polypharmacy (≥5 drugs)	Key correlates/Risk factors	References
U.S. adults ≥65 years' overall (2017–2018)	17.1%	Age, multimorbidity, race, education	[3, 4]
U.S. adults ≥65 years	45.1%	Advanced age, hypertension, diabetes, cardiovascular disease	[3, 4]
European adults ≥65 years	32.1–43.1%	Multimorbidity, frailty, healthcare utilization	[5, 6]
European adults ≥80 years	56.0%	Advanced age, frailty, cognitive impairment	[5, 6]
Long-term care residents (adults ≥65 years)	Up to 91%	Frailty, institutionalization, cognitive decline	[7]
Patients with cardiovascular disease (U.S.) adults ≥65 years	61.7%	Guideline-driven multidrug therapy	[5]
Patients in socioeconomically deprived areas (Ireland) adults ≥65 years	74.7%	Early disease onset, comorbidity clustering	[8]

**Quantitative polypharmacy is used as an epidemiological marker to identify populations at increased risk of inappropriate polypharmacy; it does not imply that all multidrug regimens are clinically inappropriate.*

Table 1.
Quantitative polypharmacy as a proxy indicator for populations at increased risk of inappropriate polypharmacy.

inappropriate polypharmacy within a broader systems-level context that encompasses prescribing practices, patient factors, and evolving healthcare technologies.

2. The clinical and economic consequences of inappropriate polypharmacy

Problematic polypharmacy has profound consequences, triggering a cascade of adverse clinical and economic outcomes. In particular, polypharmacy substantially increases the risk of drug–drug interactions (DDIs), a major mechanism and source of preventable adverse drug events (ADEs). The most immediate risks include a sharp rise in ADEs, DDIs, and drug-disease interactions. The likelihood of an ADE increases exponentially with the number of prescribed medications—outpatients taking five or more drugs face an 88% higher risk compared to those on fewer medications [6]. A prospective study of hospitalized older adults on five or more medications revealed an alarming 80% prevalence of potential DDIs mediated by the hepatic cytochrome P450 (CYP) enzyme system. These risks are far from trivial: ADEs rank among the fourth to sixth leading causes of death worldwide and account for up to 10% of hospital admissions among older adults [7, 8].

2.1 The prescribing cascade: A vicious cycle

A particularly concerning driver of inappropriate polypharmacy is the "prescribing cascade," where the side effect of one drug is misinterpreted as a new medical condition, leading to the unnecessary prescription of additional medications. This creates a vicious cycle of escalating medication burden and risk. A systematic review identified 49 distinct prescribing cascade pathways, with the most frequent stemming from cardiovascular and nervous system drugs. Classic examples include prescribing diuretics for edema caused by calcium channel blockers or antiparkinsonian agents to counteract the antipsychotic-induced extrapyramidal symptoms. Such cascades not only worsen polypharmacy but also amplify patient harm [9].

The economic burden of polypharmacy is staggering, straining healthcare systems worldwide. If healthcare systems already bear a substantial financial burden from appropriate polypharmacy—where multiple medications are clinically necessary—then the costs associated with inappropriate and unnecessary polypharmacy are even more excessive and unjustifiable.

Current data illustrate the scale of this burden: a 2022 Washington state analysis found that polypharmacy was associated with $17,733 higher annual medical costs per senior compared to those without polypharmacy. Similarly, a national study of older adults with cardiovascular disease (CVD) revealed that polypharmacy nearly doubled total healthcare expenditures—rising from $8815 to $19,068 annually—and tripled pharmacy-related spending. When these medications are inappropriate, these costs represent a complete loss of resources, stemming from preventable hospitalizations, unnecessary outpatient visits, and the direct expense of medications that offer no clinical value [10].

Beyond clinical and financial impacts, inappropriate polypharmacy severely diminishes patients' quality of life. It is strongly associated with reduced health-related quality of life (HRQOL), particularly in physical functioning, and contributes to psychological distress, medication non-adherence, and increased caregiver burden.

The cumulative effect is a healthcare paradox: While medications are prescribed to improve health, excessive and inappropriate use often leads to greater harm than benefit.

Generally, polypharmacy inevitably leads to medication non-adherence, a widespread and complex challenge in patient care. The sheer cognitive and logistical burden of managing multiple medications—each with different dosages, schedules, and administration instructions—overwhelms many patients, particularly older adults who may also contend with age-related cognitive decline, vision impairment, or dexterity limitations. Studies highlight the severity of this issue: One investigation of older adults with polypharmacy found a non-adherence rate of 79.6%, underscoring the difficulty patients face in following complex regimens [11, 12].

The root causes of non-adherence are multifaceted. Some patients simply forget to take their medications, while others struggle with the high financial cost of multiple prescriptions. Many lose confidence in their treatment, either due to unclear perceived benefits or unreported side effects that prompt them to independently adjust or discontinue medications without consulting their provider. This erratic adherence behavior contributes to treatment failure, disease progression, and avoidable hospitalizations, perpetuating a vicious cycle of escalating healthcare utilization [13, 14].

Also, the prevailing clinical paradigm often assumes that guideline-concordant, or "appropriate," polypharmacy sufficiently mitigates the risks associated with multiple medication uses; however, current evidence demonstrates that such regimens still precipitate substantial iatrogenic harm. Even when optimized according to standard care protocols, polypharmacy introduces the measurable risks driven by cumulative drug burden, unpredictable pharmacological interactions, and individual physiological vulnerabilities. For instance, patients prescribed seven or more medications face an approximate 80% risk of experiencing an adverse drug event (ADE) despite the regimen being evidence-based [15].

Furthermore, adherence to parallel, multi-disease guidelines frequently engenders clinically significant drug–drug interactions (DDIs) by design. In older adult populations with diabetes, optimized therapies still generate serious DDIs in 14–25% of cases [16], a risk mirrored broadly among older adults admitted to hospitals [17]. Similarly, DDIs account for approximately 30% of unexpected adverse events identified in spontaneous reporting systems [18]. These interactions contribute significantly to acute medical crises, including emergency department presentations driven by conflicts between baseline antihypertensives and newly prescribed acute medications [19], as well as hospital admissions in vulnerable demographics like elderly oncology patients [20, 21].

Beyond discrete interactions, the cumulative physiological burden associated with appropriate polypharmacy manifests in severe, systemic clinical outcomes. Systematic evaluations indicate that polypharmacy is linked to a pooled 18% incidence of acute kidney injury (AKI), heavily driven by the convergence of nephrotoxic agents [22]. The inherent complexity of these regimens independently increases hospital admissions for concurrent conditions, such as atrial fibrillation [23]. Moreover, even rigorously optimized regimens frequently fail to eliminate exposure to potentially inappropriate medications (PIMs). These embedded PIMs mediate a significant portion of the excess iatrogenic harm and are associated with a 30% increase in mortality among patients subject to chronic polypharmacy [24]. Consequently, the designation of a regimen as "appropriate" solely confirms its conformity to isolated evidence-based criteria; it does not guarantee the physiological capacity of multimorbid patients to safely metabolize the cumulative pharmaceutical load, underscoring the clinical necessity of targeted, patient-centered deprescribing interventions [25].

Addressing these issues require tailored interventions, such as simplified dosing schedules, medication synchronization, pill organizers, and regular medication reviews to deprescribe unnecessary drugs. Additionally, patient education, shared decision-making, and cost-reduction strategies can improve adherence and mitigate the downstream consequences of polypharmacy. Without such measures, the burden of non-adherence will continue to undermine treatment efficacy and patient outcomes.

2.2 The hidden risk: Unregulated supplements and herb-drug interactions

Compounding the challenges of prescription polypharmacy is a largely hidden and under-regulated dimension: the widespread use of herbal supplements and other complementary medicines. Driven by a desire for self-care and a common misperception that "natural" equates to "safe," patients frequently add pharmacologically active substances to their regimens without clinical oversight, creating a significant and often invisible risk of harmful herb-drug interactions (HDIs).

The risks associated with herbal supplements are magnified by a global regulatory landscape marked by profound inconsistencies, creating a false sense of security among consumers. In the United States, the Dietary Supplement Health and Education Act (DSHEA) of 1994 classifies the herbal products as dietary supplements rather than drugs, exempting manufacturers from providing the FDA with evidence of safety or efficacy before marketing. This reactive regulatory approach means action is taken only after a product is proven unsafe, allowing potentially hazardous botanical products to enter the market with minimal oversight [26].

By contrast, the European Union's Traditional Herbal Medicinal Products Directive (THMPD) requires evidence of quality, safety, and plausible efficacy for herbal products with a history of traditional use, offering greater consumer protection than the US model while still falling short of pharmaceutical standards. Asia presents a regulatory spectrum, with countries like China and India integrating some herbal products into formal medicine systems under national pharmacopeias, while others lack robust quality control and post-market surveillance. This regulatory disharmony results in dramatic variations in product quality and safety worldwide, posing significant challenges for clinicians and consumers navigating an increasingly globalized supplement market [27].

Contrary to the common perception of natural products as inherently safe, herbal supplements contain pharmacologically active compounds that interact with conventional medications through the established pharmacokinetic and pharmacodynamic mechanisms. Pharmacokinetic interactions most frequently involve modulation of the hepatic cytochrome P450 (CYP) enzyme system, which metabolize most prescription drugs. St. John's Wort serves as a prime example, acting as the potent inducer of CYP3A4, CYP1A2, and CYP2C9 isoenzymes along with P-glycoprotein, leading to accelerated metabolism and reduced efficacy of critical medications including oral contraceptives, immunosuppressants, and antiretrovirals [28, 29].

Conversely, herbs like echinacea inhibit these same enzymes, potentially elevating drug concentrations to toxic levels. Pharmacodynamic interactions occur when herbal and pharmaceutical compounds act on the same physiological pathways, as seen with the additive antiplatelet effects of garlic, ginger, and ginkgo biloba when combined with warfarin or aspirin, significantly increasing bleeding risk. Similarly, herbs like ginseng can potentiate hypoglycemic agents, while hawthorn may amplify the effects of antihypertensive medications, demonstrating that "natural" products can profoundly influence conventional drug therapy through multiple biological pathways [30, 31].

The clinical consequences of these interactions are far from theoretical, with documented cases ranging from treatment failures to life-threatening adverse events. The widespread use of herbal supplements, combined with inconsistent regulation and inadequate clinician-patient communication about their risks, creates a perfect storm for preventable medication-related harm. This situation is further complicated by the fact that many patients do not disclose herbal supplements to their healthcare providers, often because they perceive these products as harmless or fear disapproval.

The resulting information gap leaves clinicians unaware of potential interactions when prescribing medications, while consumers remain uninformed about the very real pharmacological effects of the supplements they take. Addressing this challenge requires a multi-pronged approach including improved regulatory standards, enhanced clinician education about herb-drug interactions, and open, non-judgmental communication with patients about their use of complementary therapies. Without such measures, the risks posed by herbal supplements will continue to represent an underappreciated yet significant threat to medication safety and public health.

3. A framework for intervention: Strategies for optimizing medication use

Effectively managing polypharmacy requires a multifaceted strategy that balances evidence-based prescribing with patient-centered care. The process begins with comprehensive medication review and reconciliation, a critical intervention that extends beyond merely listing prescriptions to holistically evaluating all substances a patient consumes—including prescription drugs, over-the-counter medications, and supplements—in relation to their health goals.

3.1 Comprehensive medication management and the role of the pharmacist

Comprehensive Medication Management (CMM) represents the gold standard for this approach, ensuring each medication is assessed for appropriateness, effectiveness, safety, and adherence. This continuous, patient-centered process involves identifying patients at risk, obtaining a detailed medication history, evaluating therapy, detecting drug-related problems, and developing a personalized care plan with structured follow-up [32]. Given their pharmacological expertise, clinical pharmacists play a pivotal role in leading CMM, particularly in integrated care models where they collaborate with physicians under structured agreements to adjust, initiate, or discontinue medication [33]. According to prospective study, it was shown that pharmacist-led reviews significantly improve therapy appropriateness and patient education, though the time-intensive nature of these interventions—averaging 49 minutes for initial assessments—underscores the need for dedicated clinical support [34].

3.2 Deprescribing: The systematic process of medication withdrawal

A cornerstone of polypharmacy management is deprescribing, and the systematic and supervised process of withdrawing medications when risks outweigh benefits.

This proactive approach requires careful patient assessment, identification of PIMs, prioritization based on harm-benefit ratios, and implementation of tapering regimens with close monitoring. Structured frameworks such as the ARMOR protocol and specialized resources like the Maudsley Deprescribing Guidelines provide clinicians with evidence-based methodologies for reducing medication burden [35–37]. Success hinges on shared decision-making, where clinicians and patients collaboratively align deprescribing plans with personal health priorities, emphasizing optimization rather than treatment withdrawal.

To support medication reviews and deprescribing, validated screening tools help clinicians identify inappropriate prescribing. Explicit criteria like the Beers Criteria flag high-risk medications in older adults, while the STOPP/START tool offers a more comprehensive evaluation by addressing both overprescribing and treatment gaps [38, 39]. For complex cases, implicit tools such as the Medication Appropriateness Index (MAI) enable nuanced, patient-specific assessments. The choice of tool depends on clinical context, with explicit criteria suited for rapid screening and implicit methods reserved for in-depth reviews [40].

Even the most optimized regimen fails if patients cannot adhere to it, making adherence support a critical component of polypharmacy management. Effective strategies combine education—clarifying medication purposes, benefits, and side effects—with practical interventions such as pill organizers or reminder systems. However, adherence efforts must address individual barriers, including cost, forgetfulness, or skepticism about treatment efficacy. A persistent challenge lies in reconciling disease-specific guidelines, which often promote additional medications, with holistic care models that prioritize reducing unnecessary drug burden. This tension highlights the need for clinical judgment that balances guideline-directed therapy with patient-centered priorities, such as Qol and functional status.

Implementation of context profoundly influences the success of these strategies. For example, while STOPP/START recommendations are highly effective when delivered by physicians, their impact diminishes when communicated by pharmacists—a disparity attributed to professional hierarchies rather than clinical validity. This underscores the importance of fully integrating pharmacists into care teams with defined collaborative roles to maximize their contributions. Ultimately, effective polypharmacy management demands a systematic yet flexible approach, blending structured tools with individualized care to mitigate risks while preserving the therapeutic benefits (**Table 2**).

While the theoretical foundations of Comprehensive Medication Management (CMM), deprescribing, and related pharmaceutical care strategies are the well-established, their true value lies in their demonstrated real-world impact. A critical examination of the evidence reveals a compelling yet nuanced picture: These interventions consistently excel at improving medication-related processes and generating economic value, but their ability to improve "hard" clinical endpoints such as mortality and hospitalizations present a more complex story that reflects the inherent challenges of studying frail, multimorbid populations.

The evidence supporting traditional pharmaceutical interventions is both robust and overwhelmingly positive when examining their primary targets: medication appropriateness and healthcare economics. Pharmacist-led medication reviews consistently achieve their fundamental objective of improving prescribing quality and appropriateness. Multiple studies and systematic reviews demonstrate that these interventions successfully identify and resolve medication-related problems (MRPs), including the elimination of PIMs.

Tool name	Type	Primary focus	Key strengths	Key limitations	Refs.
Beers Criteria	Explicit	Identifying PIMs in older adults.	Widely recognized, evidence-based, frequently updated by the American Geriatrics Society.	Does not address prescribing omissions; some criteria may not be applicable outside the United States.	[38, 39]
STOPP/START Criteria	Explicit	Identifying PIMs (STOPP) and Potential Prescribing Omissions (PPOs) (START).	Comprehensive, physiological systems-based approach; uniquely addresses undertreatment (omissions).	Can be complex and time-consuming due to the large number of criteria (190 in Version 3).	[38, 39]
Medication Appropriateness Index (MAI)	Implicit	Patient-specific appropriateness assessment based on 10 guiding questions.	Highly individualized and patient-centered; considers clinical complexity and context.	Time-consuming; requires a high level of clinical judgment and expertise; less standardized.	[40]

**Explicit tools apply predefined, rule-based criteria to identify potentially inappropriate prescribing, whereas implicit tools rely on individualized clinical judgment to assess medication appropriateness within the patient's specific clinical context.*

Table 2.
Comparative analysis of Key Polypharmacy Screening Tools.

A compelling example comes from a study of multidisciplinary structured medication reviews (SMRs) in care homes, which demonstrated substantial reductions in polypharmacy. The average number of medications per resident decreased from 8.32 to 6.99—a clinically meaningful reduction of 1.33 medicines per person. Notably, this included the discontinuation or modification of high-risk medications such as diuretics and anticoagulants, which are the known contributors to a significant proportion of preventable hospital admissions. Perhaps the most documented and persuasive aspect of these interventions is their economic impact. The care home SMR study projected annual net medication savings of £131,462, averaging £169 per resident [41, 42].

However, larger-scale CMM programs demonstrate even more dramatic financial benefits. A CMM program implemented across Texas primary care clinics generated an estimated $1,143,015 in cost savings through systematic resolution of drug therapy problems. Even more impressive, an analysis of a large US Medicaid plan found that CMM implementation was associated with a 19.3% decrease in total cost of care, translating to savings of $554 per patient per month. Return on investment (ROI) calculations further underscore this value proposition, with one large integrated health system reporting an impressive 12:1 ROI for its medication therapy management (MTM) program. These figures demonstrate that strategic investment in skilled clinical pharmacist time to optimize the medication use yields substantial financial returns for health systems and payers [43, 44].

Interventions focused specifically on deprescribing demonstrate similarly impressive results in reducing overall medication burden. Systematic reviews consistently conclude that deprescribing initiatives lead to statistically significant reductions in both total prescribed medications and PIMs. In one comprehensive systematic review of 14 randomized controlled trials (RCTs), 13 studies successfully demonstrated that deprescribing interventions reduced the number of drugs or doses taken by patients [45, 46].

Critically, these medication reductions are achieved with an excellent safety profile. Across the aforementioned multiple systematic reviews, researchers have found that deprescribing interventions are not associated with significant harm.

3.3 Complex outcomes: Clinical and humanistic endpoints

While the impact on medication optimization and economic measures is clearly positive, the effect of these interventions on major clinical and humanistic outcomes presents a more nuanced picture that reflects the complexity of studying vulnerable patient populations. The relationship between reducing PIMs and improving major clinical outcomes like hospitalizations, falls, and mortality is not consistently straightforward. A meta-analysis of interventions using the STOPP/START criteria found some evidence for positive clinical effects, including reduced patient falls and shorter hospital lengths of stay. However, the same analysis found no statistically significant effect on overall mortality [47]. Similarly, a comprehensive systematic review of hospital-based deprescribing interventions reached parallel conclusions; while the interventions effectively reduced PIMs, their impact on clinical outcomes like hospital readmissions and mortality remained unclear due to low-quality and highly heterogeneous available evidence [48]. Other major reviews have echoed this uncertainty, concluding that definitive evidence for consistent improvement in patient-oriented outcomes across all settings remains elusive.

Despite these mixed overall results, stronger evidence emerges for clinical benefit in specific, well-defined populations. A notable systematic review focused on older patients with life-limiting illnesses and limited life expectancy found that deprescribing dual-purpose medications (such as statins used for long-term prevention) was associated with significant mortality reduction (risk ratio of 0.59) and lower risk of acute care referrals (risk ratio of 0.40). This suggests that in end-of-life care, where therapeutic goals shift from long-term prevention to immediate QoL and symptom management, deprescribing benefits become more pronounced and clinically meaningful [48].

Evidence regarding (QoL) impact presents a similarly complex landscape. One systematic review of deprescribing RCTs reported that among five studies measuring (HRQoL) as a primary outcome, four found significant positive effects associated with the intervention. This suggests that reducing medication burden can produce tangible improvements in how patients feel and function. However, other large-scale reviews have found little to no consistent effect on QoL measures [45]. In contrast, patient satisfaction with CMM and pharmacist-led services remains consistently high, indicating that patients value the dedicated time and personalized attention these interventions provide [49].

The evidence presents a compelling paradox: interventions proven to be safe, highly effective at reducing inappropriate prescribing, and economically beneficial do not always translate into clear, consistent improvements in major health outcomes like mortality. This discrepancy does not necessarily indicate intervention failure but rather reflects several important considerations.

Many clinical trials in this field may be underpowered or have follow-up periods insufficient to detect statistically significant changes in long-term outcomes like mortality, particularly in populations with high baseline risk. A six-month follow-up period may adequately capture changes in medication counts but prove insufficient for detecting meaningful survival differences.

A "ceiling effect" may exist related to the underlying health status of target populations. Patients with the highest medication burdens are often the most severely ill and frail. While optimizing their medications represents a crucial step in reducing iatrogenic harm, it may be insufficient to fundamentally alter the trajectory of severe, complex, and often terminal illnesses. This leads to a more profound consideration: Current research may be focusing on inappropriate outcomes. For a frail, 90-year-old nursing home resident with advanced dementia, the most meaningful clinical goal may not be extending life by several months, but rather improving daily QoL by reducing sedative side effects, minimizing fall risk, and simplifying daily routines.

An intervention that successfully deprescribes a sedative hypnotic, thereby improving patient alertness and reducing fall risk, represents a clear clinical success from a patient-centered perspective. However, if that patient still gives way to their underlying end-stage disease 6 months later, a study using only mortality as its primary endpoint would incorrectly classify the intervention as "ineffective." This highlights the critical need for future research to prioritize patient-centered outcomes such as QoL, functional status, and symptom burden, which may be more sensitive to the medication optimization benefits.

This evidence landscape creates both opportunities and challenges for health system leaders. The strong and consistent data on economic benefits—demonstrated high ROI and significant cost savings—provides compelling justification for payers and administrators to invest in CMM and deprescribing programs. However, gaining broad support from frontline clinicians—who are mainly focused on improving patient care—requires a different and more targeted way of communicating.

The focus should emphasize the proven safety of these interventions, their demonstrated ability to reduce the present danger of adverse drug events, and their tangible, patient-centered benefits such as reducing side effect burden and improving QoL. While acknowledging that mortality reduction data remains evolving, the justification for these programs must be carefully tailored to resonate with the distinct priorities and motivations of different healthcare stakeholders.

The path forward requires embracing a more nuanced understanding of success—one that values both the measurable economic impact and the less quantifiable but equally important improvements in patient experience and QoL that these interventions consistently deliver.

4. The technological Frontier: Innovations in polypharmacy management and prevention

The management of polypharmacy stands at a technological inflection point. While traditional strategies remain foundational, they are often manual, time-consuming, and reactive in nature. The emergence of artificial intelligence, machine learning, and other advanced technologies promises to fundamentally reshape this landscape by offering a comprehensive suite of tools that enable proactive risk prediction, deep personalization of therapy, and enhanced patient support. These technological innovations are transforming polypharmacy management from an art of clinical judgment into a science of data-driven precision.

4.1 Next-generation clinical decision support systems

Traditional Clinical Decision Support Systems in electronic health records have long served to flag potential drug–drug interactions or contraindications. However, their utility has been significantly hampered by "alert fatigue"—these rule-based systems often generate high volumes of generic, low-relevance warnings, leading clinicians to override or ignore them and thus blunting their effectiveness. The new generation of AI-powered Clinical Decision Support Systems represents a quantum leap forward. By employing machine learning algorithms trained on vast clinical datasets, these systems can identify complex patterns and provide alerts that are more personalized, contextual, and clinically relevant, thereby reducing override rates and increasing their clinical impact [50, 51].

Several innovative platforms exemplify this transformative approach. One notable example is a commercial AI system (FeelBetter Inc., Boston, MA, USA) that analyzes comprehensive electronic health record (EHR) data to proactively identify patients at high risk of clinical deterioration due to suboptimal medication management including problematic polypharmacy. In a validation study conducted in collaboration with Brigham and Women's Hospital, a leading healthcare institution in Boston, Massachusetts, USA, the platform demonstrated exceptional performance—its medication-related warnings were accurate in 89.2% of cases and judged clinically useful by physician and pharmacist reviewers in 97.3% of cases. These AI-generated insights frequently translated into direct changes in patient care plans, such as discontinuing unnecessary dual antiplatelet-anticoagulant therapy in a patient with recent bleeding—a nuanced decision that simple rule-based alerts might miss [52].

ABiMed (developed by INSERM, France) represents another research-based Clinical Decision Support System designed to enhance rather than merely automate the medication review process. Moving beyond simple guideline checklists, it integrates multiple functions by automatically extracting and transferring patient data from general practitioners' electronic health records to pharmacists, implementing rules from guidelines like STOPP/START, and using visual analytics to present complex drug knowledge—including side effect profiles and interaction networks—in an intuitive, contextualized format. Qualitative evaluations with clinicians demonstrated high interest in this approach, which combines automated guideline execution with visual tools that support rather than replace human clinical reasoning [53].

The potential of generative AI is also being explored through large language models such as ChatGPT. Early studies testing ChatGPT's ability to make deprescribing decisions in hypothetical clinical scenarios revealed a degree of clinical nuance, with the model consistently recommending deprescribing in lower-risk patients while exercising greater caution in those with complex comorbidities like cardiovascular disease. However, significant limitations emerged: The model tended to disregard the importance of pain management, favoring discontinuation of analgesics, and its responses varied when presented with identical scenarios in different sessions. These findings highlight that while large language models show promise as potential support tools, they remain far from ready for autonomous clinical use and require extensive refinement, validation, and cautious implementation. It must be emphasized that current Large Language Models (LLMs) are not validated for autonomous clinical decision-making. Manufacturers and clinical experts alike reinforce that these tools are currently unsuitable for deprescribing decisions due to risks of "hallucination" and lack of clinical accountability [54].

Perhaps the most powerful application of AI in polypharmacy management lies in its predictive capabilities. Machine learning models can analyze millions of data points from electronic health records, insurance claims, and other sources to identify intricate patterns invisible to human analysis or simple rule-based systems. The primary function of these predictive models involves identifying patients at highest risk of polypharmacy-related harm before adverse events occur, with performance significantly surpassing traditional risk identification methods that often rely on simple medication counts.

One study demonstrated that an AI-assisted platform identified 80% of high-risk patients missed by conventional screening methods, with interventions in this AI-identified group leading to a 6% reduction in hospitalizations and a 2.6-fold decrease in adverse drug event-related emergency department visits. Another study directly compared a machine learning model against a standard polypharmacy rule of eight or more medications for predicting hospitalization. The machine learning model, incorporating multiple clinical variables, proved 3.5 times more effective at identifying patients who would subsequently require hospitalization, demonstrating vastly superior ability to target resources to those most in need [55, 56].

Machine learning is also revolutionizing drug–drug interaction prediction. Traditional approaches rely on databases of known interactions discovered through clinical trials or post-marketing surveillance. In contrast, machine learning models can predict previously unknown drug–drug interactions by training on multi-modal data including drug molecular structures, chemical properties, protein targets, and multi-omics data encompassing genomics and proteomics. Deep learning and graph neural network models can infer the likelihood of interactions between drugs that have never been studied together, transforming drug safety from a reactive to a predictive science [57, 58].

Beyond risk prediction, AI enables true personalization of treatment through sophisticated algorithms like SIENNA, a data-driven framework using contextual multi-armed bandits. This algorithm learns from treatment outcomes of large patient populations and, when presented with new patients, analyzes their specific context including demographics and comorbidities. Based on historical data from similar patients, SIENNA sequentially selects optimal medications and dosages. As an adaptive system that continuously learns and refines recommendations as more patient data becomes available, it represents a powerful, real-time approach to personalizing therapy [59, 60].

Addressing the pervasive problem of non-adherence represents another key area for technological innovation. A new generation of smart devices and mobile applications provides robust support for patients managing complex regimens. Smart devices offer active reminders and tracking to combat forgetfulness through tools like smart pill bottles and caps, such as AdhereTech's Aidia system, which use visual cues like flashing lights, auditory alerts including chimes, and text message reminders to prompt patients to take medications [61].

These devices record each bottle opening, providing objective adherence measures. Studies demonstrate their effectiveness—one trial in multiple myeloma patients found that a smart pill bottle platform improved median adherence from 87% in the control group to 100% in the intervention group. For even higher certainty levels, ingestible sensors like the ID-Cap from etectRx contain tiny sensors within capsules that, upon ingestion, send signals to wearable patches or receivers, providing definitive confirmation that medications have been taken [62, 63].

Mobile health applications are evolving from simple reminder systems into sophisticated, AI-powered health management tools. The prototype application "Polly" exemplifies this evolution by integrating AI-powered machine vision that allows patients to use their phone cameras for real-time pill verification. The app's underlying YOLOv8 computer vision model, trained to identify specific pills from images, achieved validation precision of 84.5%. This provides powerful safety checks to prevent patients from taking wrong medications—a significant risk in complex polypharmacy regimens [64, 65].

4.2 Personalization through pharmacogenomics

On the other hand, pharmacogenomics adds another layer of deep personalization by analyzing patients' unique genetic makeup to predict their responses to specific drugs. This approach shifts prescribing from "one-size-fits-all" or trial-and-error methods to precision-guided strategies. The clinical utility of pharmacogenomics lies in identifying genetic variations in key drug-metabolizing enzymes such as the cytochrome P450 family, including CYP2D6 and CYP2C19, as well as drug targets. Patients who are "poor metabolizers" for specific enzymes may be unable to break down standard drug doses processed by those enzymes, leading to drug accumulation and toxic levels causing severe side effects. Conversely, "ultra-rapid metabolizers" may clear drugs so quickly that standard doses prove ineffective [66–68].

A compelling case study illustrates this approach's power: a 66-year-old woman experiencing significant health decline with multiple falls and cognitive issues despite being on numerous medications underwent comprehensive medication review that identified several potentially inappropriate medications. A subsequent pharmacogenomic test—a simple buccal swab—revealed significant abnormalities in her CYP2D6 and CYP2C19 enzymes, meaning her body could not properly metabolize several prescribed drugs, effectively causing overdosing. Armed with this genetic information, her clinical team made evidence-based changes: Five medications were discontinued and two were replaced with alternatives not metabolized by the compromised enzymes. Results proved dramatic—within 3 months, the patient's alertness and gait improved, falls ceased, and her total medication list was reduced by 33%. This demonstrates how pharmacogenomics can uncover root causes of medication-related problems and guide highly effective, personalized deprescribing and optimization [69–71].

These technological advancements (**Table 3**) represent more than incremental improvements; they constitute a fundamental shift in polypharmacy management approaches. The true transformative potential lies not in isolated application of single technologies, but in their synergistic integration. One can envision future workflows where AI predictive models proactively identify patients at high risk for polypharmacy-related harm from electronic health record data. These patients then undergo pharmacogenomic testing, with their unique metabolic profiles integrated into health records. This combined clinical and genomic data feeds into AI-powered Clinical Decision Support Systems, providing pharmacists with highly personalized and prioritized recommendations for medication optimization and deprescribing.

This integrated approach fundamentally redefines healthcare professional roles by automating and augmenting many cognitive tasks previously performed by humans, such as risk calculation and interaction checking. This liberation allows clinicians to focus on uniquely human skills: empathy, navigating clinical ambiguity, building therapeutic alliances, and engaging in nuanced, goal-oriented patient conversations. The pharmacist's role particularly evolves from dispenser and manual reviewer to sophisticated data interpreter and clinical implementer of AI- and genomic-driven therapeutic plans. Meanwhile, patient adherence to newly optimized regimens receives support and monitoring through smart pill bottles or mobile health applications that close feedback loops by sending real-world adherence data back into systems to further refine the predictive models.

This evolution carries profound implications for future medical and pharmacy education, which must adapt to train new generations of clinicians who are not merely technology users, but skilled collaborators with intelligent systems.

AI application/ Platform	Primary function	Validated population/ Setting	Key effectiveness findings	Clinical impact
ML risk stratification platforms	Identification of high-risk patients	Older adults with multimorbidity (outpatient care)	Identified ~80% of high-risk patients missed by conventional methods	Reduced hospitalizations and ADR-related ED visits
ML hospitalization prediction models	Hospitalization risk prediction	Large outpatient cohorts with polypharmacy	3.5-fold improvement over medication count alone	Improved targeting of pharmacist interventions
FeelBetter AI-CDSS	Context-aware clinical decision support	Hospitalized and ambulatory older adults	Clinically useful alerts in 97.3% of cases	Supported deprescribing and regimen optimization
"Polly" mHealth application	Adherence support and pill verification	Older adults managing complex regimens	Pill recognition precision ~84.5%	Reduced medication errors
Smart pill bottle systems	Objective adherence monitoring	Patients receiving long-term oral therapies	Improved adherence from 87 to ~100%	Enhanced regimen persistence
Pharmacogenomics-guided medication review	Personalized deprescribing	Older adults with adverse drug reactions	Identified actionable CYP polymorphisms	Reduced medication burden and falls

Table 3.
Efficacy and validation of AI-driven polypharmacy interventions.

The transformation promises a future where technology amplifies human expertise rather than replacing it, creating more precise, personalized, and effective approaches to managing the complex challenge of polypharmacy.

5. A paradigm shift toward prevention: Rational polypharmacology and advanced drug delivery

In contrast to the reactive strategies required to manage existing polypharmacy, a proactive approach emerges from the field of drug discovery through the intentional design of multi-targeted therapies. This paradigm shift seeks to address the root cause of polypharmacy in chronic disease—multimorbidity—by building therapeutic complexity into the drug molecule itself, rather than asking patients to manage complex regimens of multiple pills.

For decades, the dominant paradigm in drug discovery was the "one-drug, one-target" model, which prized the development of highly selective molecules acting on single biological targets. While successful for many acute conditions, this approach has proven insufficient for complex, multifactorial chronic diseases like cancer, diabetes, and neurodegenerative disorders, which are driven by dysregulation across multiple interconnected pathways [72].

This recognition has given rise to the concept of rational polypharmacology, which aims at designing single chemical entities that can modulate multiple, distinct biological targets relevant to disease states. It is essential to distinguish this drug design philosophy from the patient-level problem of polypharmacy. Here, polypharmacology represents the solution: a strategy to reduce patients' pill burden and simplify treatment by consolidating multiple mechanisms of action into single molecules. The potential advantages are significant, including enhanced therapeutic efficacy through synergistic effects, the ability to use lower doses, and corresponding reductions in side effects and toxicity [73].

5.1 Advanced drug delivery: Optimizing performance and adherence

The therapeutic potential of next-generation drugs can be significantly amplified by advanced drug delivery systems (ADDS). These technologies are designed to optimize drug performance by providing sustained release, improving bioavailability, and targeting delivery to specific tissues, thereby enhancing efficacy while minimizing systemic side effects. This approach represents a fundamental shift in how drug therapy is conceptualized for complex diseases, moving beyond managing polypharmacy through patient education or adherence aids to engineering complexity out of the treatment regimen at the molecular level [74].

The most established application of the multi-targeting concept is the polypill, a fixed-dose combination of several existing medications consolidated into a single pill. Developed primarily for cardiovascular disease prevention, the polypill's rationale centers on improving adherence and simplifying the management of conditions driven by multiple risk factors such as hypertension and hyperlipidemia. Early proposed polypills typically contained a statin, several low-dose antihypertensive agents (such as ACE inhibitors, beta-blockers, and diuretics), and low-dose aspirin [75, 76].

Clinical evidence supports the benefits of the polypill approach. The landmark PolyIran trial, for example, evaluated a fixed-dose combination tablet containing aspirin, atorvastatin, hydrochlorothiazide, and either enalapril or valsartan, and reported a 34% reduction in major cardiovascular events compared with lifestyle advice alone. Although part of this benefit reflects the pharmacological effect of combining proven cardiovascular agents, the trial also demonstrated the pragmatic value of simplifying therapy—notably, improved medication adherence and greater feasibility for large-scale preventive strategies. Consistent findings from other trials have confirmed that polypills enhance long-term adherence, a critical determinant of effective chronic disease management [77, 78].

Despite compelling evidence of their efficacy, the widespread adoption of the polypill has been gradual. A significant factor in this slow uptake is the inherent inflexibility of fixed-dose combinations (FDCs), which can complicate the precise titration of individual components—a valid and essential clinical practice during the initial phases of therapy or when patients require frequent pharmacological adjustments. However, once a patient's regimen has been stabilized through individual titration, the polypill serves as a strategic solution to the challenges of polypharmacy. By consolidating stabilized doses into a single daily unit, the clinical focus shifts from managing a high "pill burden" to ensuring long-term adherence and therapeutic persistence. Consequently, the primary barrier to adoption is not the titration process itself, but the systemic failure to transition stable patients from complex multi-pill regimens to simplified, evidence-based FDCs. Beyond clinical hurdles, significant economic barriers and shifting medical guidelines continue to hinder the widespread adoption of the polypill. For instance, evolving clinical recommendations have recently questioned the role of specific components, such as aspirin for primary prevention, complicating the standardization of fixed-dose combinations (FDCs). Furthermore, in the pharmaceutical industry, the Return on Investment (ROI) for off-patent FDCs is often perceived as unfavorable. Despite being composed of generic ingredients, a new FDC is regulated as a novel drug product, necessitating the expensive clinical trials to validate safety and efficacy. This high Research and Development (R and D) expenditure, combined with a low price ceiling dictated by the cost of individual generic components, creates a unique financial disincentive. Consequently, the costs associated with complex regulatory profiling and pharmaceutical stabilization often exceed the projected market turnover, stalling the commercialization of these essential tools. Nevertheless, the polypill remains a crucial proof-of-concept, demonstrating the immense value of regimen simplification while highlighting the systemic implementation hurdles that future multi-targeted therapies must overcome [79, 80].

Recent developments aim to resolve these concerns. Modular poly-pills allow the patients to stack or interlock drug units, offering adjustable dosing while maintaining regimen simplicity. These systems have demonstrated cost-effectiveness and improved adherence in both cardiovascular and tuberculosis therapies. Fused deposition modeling (FDM) and melt-casting 3D printing techniques have enabled the development of multi-compartment tablets with customized release profiles. Examples include tablets combining immediate-release aspirin and hydrochlorothiazide with sustained-release pravastatin, atenolol, and ramipril [81–83].

The key advantage of complex emulsions in mitigating polypharmacy lies in their ability to physically segregate multiple drugs, thus preventing potential drug–drug interactions and chemical incompatibilities before administration. For instance, hydrophilic drugs can be contained within aqueous compartments while hydrophobic drugs reside in an oil phase, all within the same particle, enabling tailored drug release profiles to avoid overlapping peak plasma concentrations, or their release can be sustained over time or triggered by specific physiological stimuli such as pH or temperature. Despite their considerable promise, significant barriers hinder the widespread clinical implementation of complex emulsions. Critical challenges include ensuring long-term formulation stability, preventing the passive leakage of drugs from their compartments during storage, and, most notably, scaling up production from laboratory-scale microfluidic devices to commercially viable volumes [84].

Collectively, these advanced delivery systems facilitate the development of therapeutic platforms designed to simplify the treatment regimens. Such integrated strategies offer significant potential to reduce pill burden, improve adherence, minimize adverse effects, and enhance the pharmacoeconomic outcomes—ultimately advancing patient-centered management of multimorbid conditions.

5.2 One drug, many targets: A smart therapeutic approach

The true breakthrough of this approach lies in the design of novel multi-target-directed ligand single molecules engineered to interact with multiple, specific biological targets. This approach relocates therapeutic complexity from patients' pillboxes to medicinal chemists' laboratories. The intricate process of balancing activity at different receptors, optimizing pharmacokinetics, and minimizing off-target effects is front-loaded into the drug design phase.

This strategy is being actively pursued for diseases where combination therapy represents standard care but is often limited by pill burden and adherence challenges, particularly in neurodegeneration, oncology, and diabetes. The development of multi-target-directed ligands relies heavily on advanced technologies such as computational chemistry, artificial intelligence, and in silico modeling, which allow researchers to predict and refine compounds' multi-target profiles before undertaking laborious chemical synthesis and biological testing. Natural products, with their inherent tendency to exhibit multi-activity, serve as rich sources of chemical scaffolds and inspiration for these novel agents [85, 86].

Interestingly, targeting multiple biological pathways simultaneously can enhance therapeutic efficacy while minimizing adverse effects and drug toxicity. The convergence of diverse scientific fields, including molecular biology and medicinal chemistry, has deepened our understanding of complex disease mechanisms and accelerated the discovery of more effective treatment options.

Recent studies have highlighted the ability of various natural products such as flavonoids and other phenolic constituents—exhibit *validated multitarget biological activity*, including the concurrent inhibition or modulation of multiple disease-relevant enzymes and signaling pathways [87]. Rather than acting as nonspecific agents, these compounds exert the coordinated effects on defined molecular targets, providing a mechanistic basis for their therapeutic potential. To enhance and refine this multitarget profile, medicinal chemistry efforts have focused on structural modification and hybridization strategies, yielding optimized derivatives with improved potency and selectivity for the management of complex conditions such as neurodegenerative disorders, inflammatory diseases, and cancer [88–90]. Advances in molecular biology, network pharmacology, and systems-level analyses have further enabled the characterization of the pleiotropic mechanisms underlying these effects, revealing how single natural compounds can influence interconnected pathological pathways implicated in multifactorial disorders, including obstructive sleep apnea, diabetic complications, and drug-induced nephrotoxicity [91, 92]. Collectively, these findings suggest that, following rigorous standardization, pharmacological characterization, and comprehensive safety evaluation, selected natural products or their optimized derivatives may offer a rational means of addressing multiple therapeutic targets simultaneously. Such an approach holds potential not only for reducing reliance on multiple single-target medications—thereby mitigating inappropriate

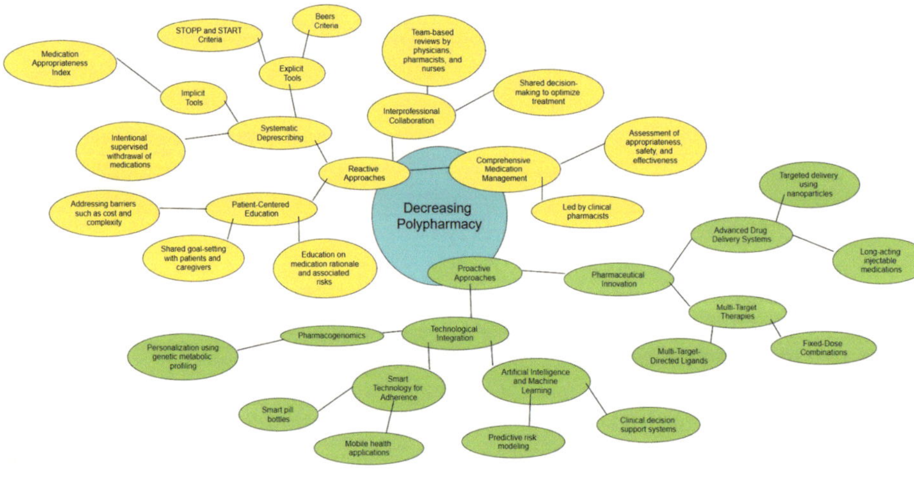

Figure 1.
Integrated approaches to reducing inappropriate polypharmacy. Yellow nodes represent clinical and organizational interventions focused on pharmacotherapy vigilance. Green nodes denote proactive strategies.

polypharmacy—but also for delivering pharmacoeconomic benefits through improved accessibility, lower cost, and simplified treatment regimens.

The success of this approach will depend not only on advances in medicinal chemistry and drug delivery technology but also on overcoming regulatory, economic, and clinical adoption challenges that have limited the widespread implementation of even relatively simple fixed-dose combinations. As these technologies mature and demonstrate clinical superiority, they promise to transform the landscape of chronic disease management by making effective polytherapy as simple as taking a single pill. **Figure 1** summarizes different strategies for mitigation and management of polypharmacy.

6. Conclusion and future perspectives

Polypharmacy represents an escalating healthcare challenge driven by aging populations and the rising prevalence of multimorbidity. Inappropriate medication use results in an increased risk of adverse drug events, complex drug–drug and drug-herb interactions, substantial financial strain on healthcare systems, and diminished patient quality of life (QoL).

Addressing this burden necessitates the widespread integration of comprehensive medication management (CMM) and systematic deprescribing into standard primary and geriatric care. While validated frameworks such as the STOPP/START criteria and the Beers list are instrumental in reducing inappropriate prescribing, the success of these interventions should be evaluated primarily through patient-centered metrics. Future research and clinical models must prioritize functional status, symptom relief, and overall QoL over traditional mortality endpoints.

The future of medication optimization relies on a proactive, data-driven paradigm. Healthcare systems must integrate artificial intelligence (AI), machine learning, and pharmacogenomics into clinical workflows to provide robust decision support and personalized risk prediction. Concurrently, pharmaceutical research should advance rational polypharmacology. Developing multi-target therapies and advanced drug delivery systems will minimize pill burden and enhance patient adherence.

Ultimately, mitigating inappropriate polypharmacy requires a coordinated, system-level response. Regulatory frameworks and reimbursement models must incentivize CMM services and facilitate the approval of multi-target therapies. Furthermore, clinical education must evolve to train healthcare professionals in utilizing digital tools, while simultaneously empowering patients to actively engage in their medication regimens. Harmonizing clinical expertise with technological innovation and supportive policy will effectively transition healthcare systems from managing the consequences of polypharmacy to actively preventing it.

Acknowledgements

The authors wish to express their deep appreciation to the *FAB-Lab for Drug Discovery from Natural Products*, Faculty of Pharmacy, Mansoura University, Egypt, for its continuous intellectual, technical, and logistical support throughout the development of this work. Founded in 1990 by Prof. Farid A. Badria, the FAB-Lab remains a leading center of excellence in pharmacognosy, integrative medicine, and translational drug discovery. Its commitment to interdisciplinary innovation and real-world impact has profoundly shaped the vision and execution of this chapter.

Abbreviations

PIMs:	potentially inappropriate medications
STOPP:	Screening Tool of Older Persons' Prescriptions
START:	Screening Tool to Alert doctors to Right Treatment
MAI:	Medication Appropriateness Index.

Author details

Farid A. Badria[1*] and Abdullah A. Elgazar[2]

1 Department of Pharmacognosy, Faculty of Pharmacy, Mansoura University, Mansoura, Egypt

2 Department of Pharmacognosy, Faculty of Pharmacy, Kafrelsheikh University, Kafrelsheikh, Egypt

*Address all correspondence to: faridbadria@gmail.com

References

[1] Tsang JY, Sperrin M, Blakeman T, Payne RA, Ashcroft D. Defining, identifying and addressing problematic polypharmacy within multimorbidity in primary care: A scoping review. BMJ Open. 2024;**14**(5):e081698

[2] Cadogan CA, Ryan C, Hughes CM. Appropriate polypharmacy and medicine safety: When many is not too many. Drug Safety. 2016;**39**:109-116

[3] Kim S, Lee H, Park J, Kang J, Rahmati M, Rhee SY, et al. Global and regional prevalence of polypharmacy and related factors, 1997-2022: An umbrella review. Archives of Gerontology and Geriatrics. 2024;**124**:105465

[4] Jokanovic N, Jamsen KM, Tan ECK, Dooley MJ, Kirkpatrick CM, Bell JS. Prevalence and variability in medications contributing to polypharmacy in long-term care facilities. Drugs - Real World Outcomes. 2017;**4**(4):235-245

[5] Wang X, Liu K, Shirai K, Tang C, Hu Y, Wang Y, et al. Prevalence and trends of polypharmacy in U.S. adults, 1999-2018. Global Health Research and Policy. 2023;**8**(1):25

[6] Bourgeois FT, Shannon MW, Valim C, Mandl KD. Adverse drug events in the outpatient setting: An 11-year national analysis. Pharmacoepidemiology and Drug Safety. 2010;**19**(9):901-910

[7] Doan J, Zakrzewski-Jakubiak H, Roy J, Turgeon J, Tannenbaum C. Prevalence and risk of potential cytochrome P450-mediated drug-drug interactions in older hospitalized patients with polypharmacy. The Annals of Pharmacotherapy. 2013;**47**(3):324-332

[8] Bonanno EG, Figueiredo T, Mimoso IF, Morgado MI, Carrilho J, Midão L, et al. Polypharmacy prevalence among older adults based on the survey of health, ageing and retirement in Europe: An update. Journal of Clinical Medicine. 2025;**14**(4):1330

[9] Chen Z, Liu Z, Zeng L, Huang L, Zhang L. Research on prescribing cascades: A scoping review. Frontiers in Pharmacology. 2023;**14**:1147921

[10] Kwak MJ, Chang M, Chiadika S, Aguilar D, Avritscher E, Deshmukh A, et al. Healthcare expenditure associated with polypharmacy in older adults with cardiovascular diseases. The American Journal of Cardiology. 2022;**169**:156-158

[11] González-Bueno J, Sevilla-Sánchez D, Puigoriol-Juvanteny E, Molist-Brunet N, Codina-Jané C, Espaulella-Panicot J. Factors associated with medication non-adherence among patients with multimorbidity and polypharmacy admitted to an intermediate care center. International Journal of Environmental Research and Public Health. 2021;**18**(18):9606

[12] Liu J, Yu Y, Yan S, Zeng Y, Su S, He T, et al. Risk factors for self-reported medication adherence in community-dwelling older patients with multimorbidity and polypharmacy: A multicenter cross-sectional study. BMC Geriatrics. 2023;**23**(1):75

[13] Kardas P. From non-adherence to adherence: Can innovative solutions resolve a longstanding problem? European Journal of Internal Medicine. 2024;**119**:6-12

[14] Arshed M, Umer MF, Kiran M, Akhter AM, Gillani AH, Qamer S, et al.

Prevalence and associated factors of non-adherence to antihyperlipidemic medication: A nationwide cross sectional survey in Pakistan. Scientific Reports. 2024;**14**(1):20613

[15] Hama J, Aziz TA, Mahwi TO, Hussen NH, Aziz DF. The Relation between Polypharmacy, Potentially Inappropriate Medications, Organ Function, and Quality of Life in Elderly Patients with Type 2 Diabetes. Hospital Pharmacy [Internet]; 2025. Available from: https://pmc.ncbi.nlm.nih.gov/articles/PMC12069312/

[16] Lu L, Wang S, Chen J, Yang Y, Wang K, Zheng J, et al. Associated adverse health outcomes of polypharmacy and potentially inappropriate medications in community-dwelling older adults with diabetes. Frontiers in Pharmacology. 2023;**14**:1284287

[17] Očovská Z, Maříková M, Vlček J. Potentially clinically significant drug-drug interactions in older patients admitted to the hospital: A cross-sectional study. Frontiers in Pharmacology. 2023;**14**:1088900

[18] Noguchi Y, Tachi T, Teramachi H. Review of statistical methodologies for detecting drug–drug interactions using spontaneous reporting systems. Frontiers in Pharmacology. 2019;**10**:1319

[19] Lilia Edith LE, Osorio García MA, Delgadillo Guzmán D, Castillo Maldonado I, Corvera Aispuro CE. Pharmacological interactions between antihypertensive regimens and drugs prescribed in the emergency department. Annales Pharmaceutiques Françaises. 2025;**83**(6):1130-1138

[20] Albayrak A, Erbay B, Kayıkçıoğlu E. Assessment of polypharmacy, potentially inappropriate medications, and drug-drug interactions in older patients with cancer. Journal of Oncology Pharmacy Practice. 2025;**31**(5):693-699

[21] Turner JP, McKinnon RA, Bell JS. The management of polypharmacy in people with cancer and chronic conditions. In: Cancer and Chronic Conditions: Addressing the Problem of Multimorbidity in Cancer Patients and Survivors. Singapore: Springer; 2016. pp. 261-286

[22] Yang F, Zhu L, Cao B, Miao H, Zeng L, Yuan Z, et al. Incidence and risk factors of acute kidney injury in patients with polypharmacy: A systematic review and meta-analysis. International Journal of Clinical Pharmacy. 2025;**47**(6):1609-1621

[23] Martinez-Montesinos L, Rivera-Caravaca JM, Agewall S, Soler E, Lip GYH, Marin F, et al. Polypharmacy and adverse events in atrial fibrillation: Main cause or reflection of multimorbidity? Biomedicine & Pharmacotherapy. 2023;**158**:114064

[24] Costanzo S, Di Castelnuovo A, Panzera T, De Curtis A, Falciglia S, Persichillo M, et al. Polypharmacy in older adults: The hazard of hospitalization and mortality is mediated by potentially inappropriate prescriptions, findings from the Moli-sani study. International Journal of Public Health. 2024;**69**:1607682

[25] Davis LE, Moen C, Glover JJ, Pogge EK. Understanding medication use behaviors and perspectives in an older cardiovascular patient population: Opportunities for patient-centered deprescribing. American Heart Journal Plus: Cardiology Research and Practice. 2022;**17**:100164

[26] Starr RR. Too little, too late: Ineffective regulation of dietary supplements in the United States.

American Journal of Public Health. 2015;**105**(3):478-485

[27] Blaze J. A comparison of current regulatory frameworks for nutraceuticals in Australia, Canada, Japan, and the United States. Innovations in Pharmacy. 2021;**12**(2):1-8

[28] Izzo AA, Ernst E. Interactions between herbal medicines and prescribed drugs: An updated systematic review. Drugs. 2009;**69**:1777-1798

[29] Chen X-W, Sneed KB, Pan S-Y, Cao C, Kanwar JR, Chew H, et al. Herb-drug interactions and mechanistic and clinical considerations. Current Drug Metabolism. 2012;**13**(5):640-651

[30] Hansen TS, Nilsen OG. Echinacea purpurea and P-glycoprotein drug transport in Caco-2 cells. Phytotherapy Research: An International Journal Devoted to Pharmacological and Toxicological Evaluation of Natural Product Derivatives. 2009;**23**(1):86-91

[31] Freeman C, Spelman K. A critical evaluation of drug interactions with Echinacea spp. Molecular Nutrition & Food Research. 2008;**52**(7):789-798

[32] Ramalho de Oliveira D, Brummel AR, Miller DB. Medication therapy management: 10 years of experience in a large integrated health care system. Journal of Managed Care Pharmacy. 2010;**16**(3):185-195

[33] Isetts BJ, Schondelmeyer SW, Artz MB, Lenarz LA, Heaton AH, Wadd WB, et al. Clinical and economic outcomes of medication therapy management services: The Minnesota experience. Journal of the American Pharmacists Association. 2008;**48**(2):203-214

[34] Castelli G, Bacci J, Dombrowski S, Osborne M, Difilippo A, Klatt P, et al. Pharmacist-delivered comprehensive medication management within family medicine practices an evaluation of the SCRIPT project. Family Medicine. 2018;**50**(8):605-612

[35] Reeve E, Gnjidic D, Long J, Hilmer S. A systematic review of the emerging definition of 'deprescribing' with network analysis: Implications for future research and clinical practice. British Journal of Clinical Pharmacology. 2015;**80**(6):1254-1268

[36] Haque R. ARMOR: A tool to evaluate polypharmacy in elderly persons. Annals of Long-Term Care. 2009;**17**(6):26-30

[37] Scott IA, Hilmer SN, Reeve E, Potter K, Le Couteur D, Rigby D, et al. Reducing inappropriate polypharmacy: The process of deprescribing. JAMA Internal Medicine. 2015;**175**(5):827-834

[38] O'Mahony D, O'Sullivan D, Byrne S, O'Connor MN, Ryan C, Gallagher P. STOPP/START criteria for potentially inappropriate prescribing in older people: Version 2. Age and Ageing. 2014;**44**(2):213-218

[39] American Geriatrics Society Beers Criteria® Update Expert P. American Geriatrics Society 2023 updated AGS Beers Criteria® for potentially inappropriate medication use in older adults. Journal of the American Geriatrics Society. 2023;**71**(7):2052-2081

[40] Hanlon JT, Schmader KE, Samsa GP, Weinberger M, Uttech KM, Lewis IK, et al. A method for assessing drug therapy appropriateness. Journal of Clinical Epidemiology. 1992;**45**(10):1045-1051

[41] Radcliffe E, Saucedo AR, Howard C, Sheikh C, Bradbury K, Rutter P, et al. Development of a complex multidisciplinary medication review

and deprescribing intervention in primary care for older people living with frailty and polypharmacy. PLoS One. 2025;**20**(4):e0319615

[42] Marchant R, Thorman E, Page E, Worth C, Allcock D, Fraser H, et al. 1607 multidisciplinary structured medication review reduces inappropriate polypharmacy and associated costs in care homes. Age and Ageing. 2023;**52**(Supplement_2):afad104-013

[43] Brummel A, Lustig A, Westrich K, Evans MA, Plank GS, Penso J, et al. Best practices: Improving patient outcomes and costs in an ACO through comprehensive medication therapy management. Journal of Managed Care & Specialty Pharmacy. 2014;**20**(12):1152-1158

[44] Chung TH, Hernandez RJ, Libaud-Moal A, Nguyen LK, Lal LS, Swint JM, et al. The evaluation of comprehensive medication management for chronic diseases in primary care clinics, a Texas delivery system reform incentive payment program. BMC Health Services Research. 2020;**20**(1):671

[45] Omuya H, Nickel C, Wilson P, Chewning B. A systematic review of randomised-controlled trials on deprescribing outcomes in older adults with polypharmacy. The International Journal of Pharmacy Practice. 2023;**31**(4):349-368

[46] Chua S, Todd A, Reeve E, Smith SM, Fox J, Elsisi Z, et al. Deprescribing interventions in older adults: An overview of systematic reviews. PLoS One. 2024;**19**(6):e0305215

[47] Hill-Taylor B, Walsh K, Stewart S, Hayden J, Byrne S, Sketris IS, et al. Effectiveness of the STOPP/START (screening tool of older persons' potentially inappropriate prescriptions/ screening tool to alert doctors to the right treatment) criteria: Systematic review and meta-analysis of randomized controlled studies. Journal of Clinical Pharmacy and Therapeutics. 2016;**41**(2):158-169

[48] Thillainadesan J, Gnjidic D, Green S, Hilmer SN. Impact of deprescribing interventions in older hospitalised patients on prescribing and clinical outcomes: A systematic review of randomised trials. Drugs & Aging. 2018;**35**:303-319

[49] Pestka DL, Sorge LA, Mendkoff J, Frail CK, Funk KA, Carroll JK, et al. Assessing the state of comprehensive medication management in a sample of primary care clinics. Innovations in Pharmacy. 2019;**10**(1):10-24926

[50] McCoy AB, Thomas EJ, Krousel-Wood M, Sittig DF. Clinical decision support alert appropriateness: A review and proposal for improvement. Ochsner Journal. 2014;**14**(2):195-202

[51] Gomez-Cabello CA, Borna S, Pressman S, Haider SA, Haider CR, Forte AJ. Artificial-intelligence-based clinical decision support systems in primary care: A scoping review of current clinical implementations. European Journal of Investigation in Health, Psychology and Education [Internet]. 2024;**14**(3):685-698

[52] Seger DL, Amato MG, Frits M, Iannaccone C, Mugal A, Chang F, et al. A machine learning technology for addressing medication-related risk in older, multimorbid patients. The American Journal of Managed Care. 2024;**30**(8):e233-e239

[53] Abdelmalek M, Romain L, Nada B, Thibaud L, Yoann LB, Christian S, et al. ABiMed: An intelligent and visual clinical decision support system for medication reviews and polypharmacy management. BMC Medical Informatics and Decision Making. 2025;**25**(1):173

[54] Aydin S, Karabacak M, Vlachos V, Margetis K. Navigating the potential and pitfalls of large language models in patient-centered medication guidance and self-decision support. Frontiers in Medicine. 2025;**12**:1527864

[55] Hartshorne J. Polypharmacy, artificial intelligence (AI) and rational medication prescribing-the new Frontier. International Dentistry-African Edition. 2023;**13**(6):32-40

[56] Hefti E, Xie Y, Engelen K. Machine learning model better identifies patients for pharmacist intervention to reduce hospitalization risk in a large outpatient population. Journal of Medical Artificial Intelligence. 2025;**8**:11

[57] Ryu JY, Kim HU, Lee SY. Deep learning improves prediction of drug–drug and drug–food interactions. Proceedings of the National Academy of Sciences. 2018;**115**(18):E4304-E4E11

[58] Han K, Cao P, Wang Y, Xie F, Ma J, Yu M, et al. A review of approaches for predicting drug–drug interactions based on machine learning. Frontiers in Pharmacology. 2022;**12**:814858

[59] Baig MM, Hobson C, GholamHosseini H, Ullah E, Afifi S. Generative AI in improving personalized patient care plans: Opportunities and barriers towards its wider adoption. Applied Sciences [Internet]. 2024;**14**(23):10899

[60] Banumathi K, Venkatesan L, Benjamin LS, Vijayalakshmi K, Satchi NS. Reinforcement learning in personalized medicine: A comprehensive review of treatment optimization strategies. Cureus. 2025;**17**(4):e82756

[61] Mauro J, Mathews KB, Sredzinski ES. Effect of a smart pill bottle and pharmacist intervention on medication adherence in patients with multiple myeloma new to lenalidomide therapy. Journal of Managed Care & Specialty Pharmacy. 2019;**25**(11):1244-1254

[62] Faisal S, Samoth D, Aslam Y, Patel H, Park S, Baby B, et al. Key features of smart medication adherence products: Updated scoping review. JMIR Aging. 2023;**6**:e50990

[63] Peng Y, Wang H, Fang Q, Xie L, Shu L, Sun W, et al. Effectiveness of mobile applications on medication adherence in adults with chronic diseases: A systematic review and meta-analysis. Journal of Managed Care & Specialty Pharmacy. 2020;**26**(4):550-561

[64] Messner E-M, Probst T, O'Rourke T, Stoyanov S, Baumeister H. mHealth applications: Potentials, limitations, current quality and future directions. In: Baumeister H, Montag C, editors. Digital Phenotyping and Mobile Sensing: New Developments in Psychoinformatics. Cham: Springer International Publishing; 2019. pp. 235-248

[65] Alahmadi T, Alsaedi R, Alfadli A, Alzubaidi O, Aldhahri A. A computer vision-based pill recognition application: Bridging gaps in medication understanding for the elderly. International Journal of Advanced Computer Science & Applications. 2024;**15**(7):698-705

[66] Roberts B, Cooper Z, Lu S, Stanley S, Majda BT, Collins KRL, et al. Utility of pharmacogenetic testing to optimise antidepressant pharmacotherapy in youth: A narrative literature review. Frontiers in Pharmacology. 2023;**14**:1267294

[67] Qahwaji R, Ashankyty I, Sannan NS, Hazzazi MS, Basabrain AA, Mobashir M. Pharmacogenomics: A genetic approach to drug development and therapy. Pharmaceuticals. 2024;**17**(7):940

[68] Aneesh TP, Sonal Sekhar M, Asha A, Chandran L, Zachariah SM. Pharmacogenomics: The right drug to the right person. Journal of Clinical Medicine Research [Internet]. 2009;**0**(4):191-194. Available from: https://www.jocmr.org/index.php/JOCMR/article/view/207/109

[69] Brockmöller J, Stingl JC. Multimorbidity, polypharmacy and pharmacogenomics in old age. Pharmacogenomics. 2017;**18**(6):515-517

[70] Just KS, Schneider KL, Schurig M, Stingl JC, Brockmöller J. Falls: The adverse drug reaction of the elderly and the impact of pharmacogenetics. Pharmacogenomics. 2017;**18**(13):1281-1297

[71] Trenaman SC, Bowles SK, Andrew MK, Goralski K. The role of sex, age and genetic polymorphisms of CYP enzymes on the pharmacokinetics of anticholinergic drugs. Pharmacology Research & Perspectives. 2021;**9**(3):e00775

[72] Shaaban AE, Ali AR, Ayyad SN, Badria FA. Multi-target directed ligands inspired natural products as an effective approach for the treatment of complex chronic health disorders. Bioorganic Chemistry. 2025;**154**:108075

[73] Löscher W. Single-target versus multi-target drugs versus combinations of drugs with multiple targets: Preclinical and clinical evidence for the treatment or prevention of epilepsy. Frontiers in Pharmacology. 2021;**12**:730257

[74] Crommelin DJA, Florence AT. Towards more effective advanced drug delivery systems. International Journal of Pharmaceutics. 2013;**454**(1):496-511

[75] Lonn E, Bosch J, Teo KK, Pais P, Xavier D, Yusuf S. The polypill in the prevention of cardiovascular diseases: Key concepts, current status, challenges, and future directions. Circulation. 2010;**122**(20):2078-2088

[76] Castellano JM, Sanz G, Peñalvo JL, Bansilal S, Fernández-Ortiz A, Alvarez L, et al. A polypill strategy to improve adherence: Results from the FOCUS project. Journal of the American College of Cardiology. 2014;**64**(20):2071-2082

[77] Roshandel G, Khoshnia M, Poustchi H, Hemming K, Kamangar F, Gharavi A, et al. Effectiveness of polypill for primary and secondary prevention of cardiovascular diseases (PolyIran): A pragmatic, cluster-randomised trial. The Lancet. 2019;**394**(10199):672-683

[78] Baumgartner A, Drame K, Geutjens S, Airaksinen M. Does the polypill improve patient adherence compared to its individual formulations? A systematic review. Pharmaceutics. 2020;**12**(2):190

[79] Webster R, Castellano JM, Onuma OK. Putting polypills into practice: Challenges and lessons learned. The Lancet. 2017;**389**(10073):1066-1074

[80] Yusuf S, Pinto FJ. The polypill: From concept and evidence to implementation. Lancet (London, England). 2022;**400**(10364):1661-1663

[81] Mazarura KR, Pradeep K, Choonara YE. Customized 3D printed multi-drug systems: An effective and efficient approach to polypharmacy. Expert Opinion on Drug Delivery. 2022;**19**(9):1149-1163

[82] Karavasili C, Babaee S, Kutty S, Chu JN, Min S, Fitzgerald N, et al. Modular titratable polypills for personalized medicine and simplification of complex medication regimens. Advanced Healthcare Materials. 2023;**12**(27):2301101

[83] Khaled SA, Burley JC, Alexander MR, Yang J, Roberts CJ. 3D printing of five-in-one dose combination polypill with defined immediate and sustained release profiles. Journal of Controlled Release. 2015;**217**:308-314

[84] Orlu-Gul M, Topcu AA, Shams T, Mahalingam S, Edirisinghe M. Novel encapsulation systems and processes for overcoming the challenges of polypharmacy. Current Opinion in Pharmacology. 2014;**18**:28-34

[85] Rafehi M, Möller M, Ismail Al-Khalil W, Stefan SM. Medicinal polypharmacology in the clinic - Translating the polypharmacolome into therapeutic benefit. Pharmaceutical Research. 2024;**41**(3):411-417

[86] Anighoro A, Bajorath J, Rastelli G. Polypharmacology: Challenges and opportunities in drug discovery: Miniperspective. Journal of Medicinal Chemistry. 2014;**57**(19):7874-7887

[87] Omar RM, Badria FA, Galala AA. An emerging flavone glycoside from *Phyllanthus emblica* L.: A promiscuous enzyme inhibitor and potential therapeutic in chronic diseases. South African Journal of Botany. 2023;**153**:290-296

[88] Shaaban AE, Ali AR, Ayyad SN, Badria FA. Unveiling the potential of novel natural product-based MTDLs that integrate cinnamamide scaffold as multifunctional agents for the treatment of Alzheimer's disease. Bioorganic Chemistry. 2025;**163**:108666

[89] El Hamaky NFM, Hamdi A, Bayoumi WA, Elgazar AA, Nasr MNA. Novel quinazolin-2-yl 1,2,3-triazole hybrids as promising multi-target anticancer agents: Design, synthesis, and molecular docking study. Bioorganic Chemistry. 2024;**148**:107437

[90] Adawy HA, Tawfik SS, Elgazar AA, Selim KB, Goda FE. Design, synthesis, and in vitro and in vivo biological evaluation of triazolopyrimidine hybrids as multitarget directed anticancer agents. RSC Advances. 2024;**14**(48):35239-35254

[91] Abass SA, Elgazar AA, El-Kholy SS, El-Refaiy AI, Nawaya RA, Bhat MA, et al. Unraveling the nephroprotective potential of papaverine against cisplatin toxicity through mitigating oxidative stress and inflammation: Insights from in silico, in vitro, and in vivo investigations. Molecules. 2024;**29**(9):1927

[92] Sharawi ZW, Abass SA, Zubair MA, Hegazy RA, Farrag FA, Hamdi A, et al. Khellin mitigates cisplatin-induced renal injury by targeting oxidative stress, inflammation, and apoptosis: Integration of network pharmacology, molecular docking, and preclinical validation. Pharmaceuticals. 2025;**18**(6):836

Chapter 3

Medication Safety in Maternal Care: Addressing Inappropriate Prescribing during Pregnancy and Lactation

Giada Crescioli, Costanza Cacini, Roberto Bonaiuti and Alfredo Vannacci

Abstract

Medication use during pregnancy and lactation presents unique clinical challenges due to the profound physiological changes of the maternal body and the potential risks to fetal and neonatal health. This chapter examines the prevalence and clinical implications of pharmacological treatments in maternal care, with particular attention to inappropriate prescribing practices and their consequences. It highlights the principles of rational prescribing and the role of deprescribing strategies in minimizing harm and optimizing therapeutic outcomes. Core topics include pharmacokinetics in pregnancy, teratogenic and neonatal risks, drug safety classification systems, and lactation-related considerations. Emphasis is placed on the importance of pharmacovigilance, individualized care, and the use of evidence-based resources to guide clinical decisions. By integrating current guidelines with clinical reasoning, the chapter supports a safer, more informed approach to pharmacological management in pregnant and breastfeeding women.

Keywords: pregnancy, lactation, medication safety, inappropriate medication use, prescribing practices

1. Introduction

Perinatal medicine and pharmacology focus on the health and well-being of both the mother and the child throughout all stages of pregnancy—from conception to childbirth—and during the first year after birth.

The World Health Organization (WHO) defines perinatal health as the well-being of women during pregnancy, childbirth, and the postnatal period. A key WHO goal is to ensure access to respectful, high-quality care to support the health of both mothers and newborns. Despite its importance and a 38% reduction in related deaths by 2019, access to perinatal care remains unequal, and overall progress is still limited [1].

In this field, research in pharmacology, pharmacovigilance, and pharmacoepidemiology plays a critical role, especially when conditions associated with adverse pregnancy outcomes can be effectively treated using available medications [2]. Mothers are commonly exposed to drugs during pregnancy, at birth, or in the postpartum period, and exposure to pharmacological therapies has increased in recent years [3]. However, current knowledge regarding the safe and appropriate use of medicines in pregnant and breastfeeding women remains limited. This is partly due to the historical exclusion of women of childbearing age from clinical trials, as well as the observational nature of many studies on this topic [4]. Similarly, inappropriate prescribing and deprescribing may pose a significant risk both to the mother and children, and effective risk communication and careful benefit–risk assessment are essential [5].

This chapter will explore the key characteristics that make pregnant and breastfeeding women a population requiring special consideration. It will begin with an overview of pharmacokinetic and pharmacodynamic changes during pregnancy, examine current data on medication use, define the risks of teratogenicity, embryotoxicity, and fetotoxicity, review major drug classification systems for use during pregnancy and lactation, and evaluate the benefit/risk profiles of commonly prescribed drug classes in this population.

2. Maternal physiology and pharmacokinetics

Pregnancy is a particularly delicate phase in a woman's life, during which numerous anatomical and physiological changes occur to meet increased metabolic demands. These adaptations involve all major body systems [6].

The heart is displaced upwards and to the left due to the elevated diaphragm, and the left ventricle enlarges to accommodate greater blood volume. Cardiac output increases from early gestation and peaks during the third trimester [7]. Blood pressure initially decreases, reaching its lowest point between the 24th and 26th weeks, then gradually rises again, while plasma volume expands significantly to meet the demands of the placenta and the fetus [8]. This increase in plasma volume affects drug pharmacokinetics by increasing the apparent volume of distribution, especially for hydrophilic drugs. Furthermore, maternal plasma concentrations of albumin and α1-acid glycoprotein decrease, resulting in a higher proportion of free (active) drug in circulation [6].

In the gastrointestinal tract, nausea and vomiting—often beginning in the second week of pregnancy and possibly lasting into the third trimester—can compromise drug absorption [9]. Elevated levels of progesterone and estrogen also slow gastric emptying, particularly in early pregnancy, delaying peak plasma concentrations of drugs. Metabolic activity is altered as well: high levels of progesterone induce several phase I and phase II enzymes, including cytochrome P450 isoforms (CYP2D6, 2A6, 2C9, 3A4) and uridine 5′-diphospho-glucuronosyltransferase (UGT1A1), increasing the metabolic clearance of many pharmacologically active substances [10, 11].

Carbohydrate and lipid metabolism also undergo significant changes. Despite increased insulin secretion due to pancreatic β-cell hyperplasia, pregnant women develop relative insulin resistance, associated with elevated postprandial glucose levels [12]. This condition is driven by increased secretion of placental lactogen, growth hormone, progesterone, cortisol, and prolactin. The resulting relative hypoglycemia triggers lipolysis, allowing the mother to rely more on fatty acids as an energy source, preserving glucose and amino acids for fetal use. If pancreatic function is insufficient, gestational diabetes may occur, which typically resolves postpartum [13].

The respiratory system adapts to increased oxygen requirements through hyperventilation, resulting in elevated arterial pO_2, decreased pCO_2, and a reduction in serum bicarbonate. In late pregnancy, diaphragmatic movement is restricted due to its upward displacement. As a result, some women may experience mild dyspnea at rest, which often improves with light activity [14].

Due to the increasing plasma volume, the glomerular filtration rate (GFR) rises by approximately 50%. The hormone relaxin promotes renal vasodilation by stimulating endothelin production, which in turn induces nitric oxide (NO) synthesis [15]. This reduction in vascular resistance offsets the marked increase in renal plasma flow, maintaining stable glomerular hydrostatic pressure. Kidney size increases by 1–1.5 cm, and mechanical pressure on the ureters leads to dilation of the renal pelvis and calyces. Progesterone helps mitigate these anatomical changes by reducing ureteral tone and peristalsis [16].

2.1 Fetal-to-maternal drug ratio (F/M ratio)

Given the many physiological changes from conception through postpartum, pharmacological research has focused on studying drug pharmacokinetics during pregnancy and lactation. The objective is to optimize therapy and establish appropriate dosing regimens that ensure a favorable risk–benefit ratio for both mother and fetus [17].

A major area of investigation involves the transplacental transfer of drugs and their passage into breast milk. Common methodologies include measurement of drug concentrations in umbilical cord blood, animal models (though often limited in translatability), *ex vivo* perfusion of human placental cotyledons, and, more recently, physiologically-based pharmacokinetic (PBPK) models [18].

Studying maternal-fetal drug transfer is crucial to identifying potential adverse effects on the developing fetus and has led to the classification of substances with teratogenic and/or fetotoxic properties. The fetal-to-maternal (F/M) ratio reflects the relative concentration of substances in the fetal and maternal bloodstream and is useful for assessing how compounds cross the placenta and affect fetal development [19]. Drug transfer is enhanced for small molecules (molecular weight < 600 Da) with high lipid solubility. In contrast, strong binding to maternal plasma proteins—especially albumin—reduces placental transfer. Weak bases may become trapped in the more acidic fetal circulation. Additionally, the placenta contains various membrane transporters, such as ATP-binding cassette (ABC) transporters like P-glycoprotein (P-gp). Efflux transporters on the maternal-facing side of the syncytiotrophoblast limit fetal exposure, while transporters on the fetal-facing side may facilitate drug transfer. Genetic polymorphisms in these transporters can significantly influence placental drug permeability [20]. **Table 1** and **Figure 1** outline the key maternal adaptations across different organ systems that occur during pregnancy and highlight how these changes influence drug pharmacokinetics and pharmacodynamics. Understanding these modifications is essential for optimizing drug dosing and ensuring maternal-fetal safety.

3. Teratogenicity and effects of drug exposure in neonates

The passage of pharmacological agents from the maternal to the fetal circulation is a crucial determinant of fetal exposure and potential harm. Understanding the nature and timing of exposure is essential to assessing the risk of congenital anomalies, neonatal toxicity, and long-term developmental effects.

System	Changes	Pharmacological implication
Cardiovascular	↑ Cardiac output, ↓ blood pressure, ↑ plasma volume	↑ Volume of distribution, ↓ plasma drug concentrations for hydrophilic compounds; higher doses may be needed
Plasma protein binding	↓ Albumin and α1-acid glycoprotein	↑ Free (active) drug fraction → potentially increased efficacy or toxicity
Gastrointestinal	Nausea, vomiting, delayed gastric emptying	↓ Absorption and delayed time to peak plasma concentration
Hepatic metabolism	↑ CYP enzymes (2D6, 2A6, 2C9, 3A4) and UGT1A1 activity	↑ Drug clearance, ↓ half-life of metabolized drugs
Glucose and lipid metabolism	↑ Insulin resistance, ↑ lipolysis due to hormonal changes	Risk of gestational diabetes; altered response to antidiabetic drugs
Respiratory	↑ Ventilation, ↓ pCO_2, ↑ pO_2	Changes in acid–base balance may affect drug pharmacodynamics
Renal	↑ GFR, ↑ renal plasma flow, kidney enlargement	↑ Renal clearance of hydrophilic drugs, ↓ half-life
Placental drug transfer	Dependent on molecular weight, lipophilicity, protein binding, ionization	Small, lipophilic, poorly protein-bound drugs cross more easily; weak bases may accumulate in fetal circulation
Placental transporter (i.e., P-gp)	Drug efflux (maternal side) or influx (fetal side); affected by transporter location and genetic polymorphisms	Modulate fetal drug exposure; polymorphisms may increase or decrease placental drug transfer

Table 1.
Summary of the major physiological changes during pregnancy and their pharmacological implications.

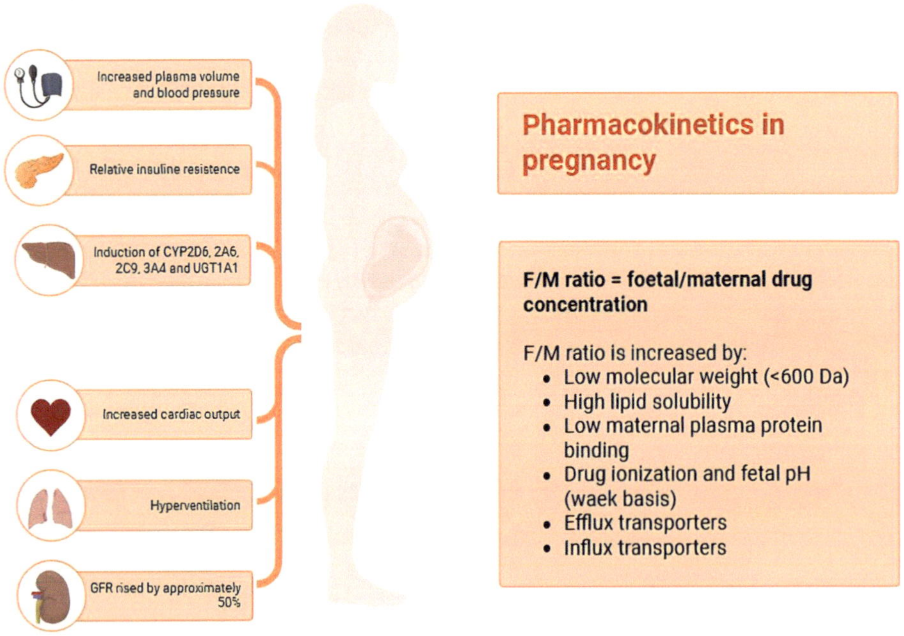

Figure 1.
Pharmacokinetic mechanisms modulating fetal exposure to maternal drugs.

Teratogenicity and fetotoxicity are distinct yet related concepts. *Teratogenicity* refers to structural or functional defects in the developing embryo caused by exposure to external agents during organogenesis, while *fetotoxicity* includes toxic effects on fetal organs and systems occurring at later stages of gestation [21]. Although only a limited number of drugs are proven human teratogens, the lack of rigorous data in pregnant populations necessitates cautious prescribing and post-market surveillance.

3.1 Teratogenicity: Definition, critical timing (e.g., embryonic vs. fetal period)

Teratogens are agents that disrupt normal embryonic development, leading to congenital malformations, miscarriage, or functional deficits. Among the best-known therapeutic drugs with established teratogenic effects are inhibitors of the renin–angiotensin system, thalidomide, isotretinoin, warfarin, valproic acid, and carbamazepine, and therefore their use is strictly inappropriate during pregnancy [21]. The sensitivity to teratogenic effects is highly time-dependent, with the most critical period being the embryonic phase (weeks 3–8 postconception), during which organogenesis occurs [22]. Exposure to teratogens during this window can cause major structural anomalies.

- *Preimplantation period (0–2 weeks)*: typically results in an "all-or-nothing" effect, with either embryonic death or full recovery;

- *Embryonic period (3–8 weeks)*: highest susceptibility to major malformations (e.g., neural tube defects, limb deformities, cardiac anomalies);

- *Fetal period (9 weeks to term)*: Risk shifts to growth retardation, minor anomalies, or functional abnormalities (e.g., neurodevelopmental delay, endocrine disruption).

Timing, dose, duration, route of administration, and fetal genetic susceptibility all influence drug-related teratogenicity. For example, valproic acid, when used during early pregnancy, is strongly associated with neural tube defects, whereas angiotensin-converting enzyme (ACE) inhibitors can induce fetal renal damage if used in the second or third trimester. **Table 2** presents selected examples of drugs with known teratogenic potential that should therefore be avoided during pregnancy, based on both preclinical studies and human data. For each compound, observed effects in animal models and documented outcomes in human pregnancies are reported, along with the critical window of exposure (defined as the gestational period during which the risk of adverse developmental effects is highest).

3.2 Neonatal effects: Toxicity, withdrawal syndromes, developmental impact

Neonatal complications may arise from direct toxicity, withdrawal syndromes, or long-term developmental disturbances (all of which warrant close clinical attention) [24].

Some drugs can cause acute toxicity in the newborn, particularly when administered late in pregnancy or intrapartum. For instance, opioids and benzodiazepines are known to depress respiratory drive in neonates, sometimes requiring ventilatory support. Their use during labor should be deeply evaluated by healthcare professionals, and only if the benefits outweigh the risks. Certain antibiotics, such as sulfonamides, may displace bilirubin from albumin binding sites, increasing the risk

Drug	Observed Effects in Animal Studies	Observed Effects in Humans	Critical Window
Valproic acid	Exencephaly in hamsters and mice	Neural tube defects (e.g., spina bifida), facial dysmorphism	Weeks 3–4 (neural tube closure)
ACE inhibitors	Fetal loss in sheep and rabbits	Renal dysgenesis, hypocalvaria, skull ossification defects	2nd-3rd trimester
Carbamazepine	Cleft palate, growth delay, dilated ventricles in mice	Neural tube defects, craniofacial anomalies	Weeks 3–6
Phenytoin	Cleft palate, renal, and CNS defects in rodents	Fetal hydantoin syndrome (growth delay, facial anomalies, limb defects)	1st trimester
Warfarin	Skeletal malformations, maxillonasal hypoplasia in rats	Fetal warfarin syndrome: nasal hypoplasia, stippled epiphyzes, CNS defects	Weeks 6–9
Isotretinoin	CNS and cardiovascular malformations in rats and rabbits	Retinoid embryopathy: craniofacial defects, heart anomalies, thymic hypoplasia	Weeks 3–5
Thalidomide	Limb-reduction defects in rabbits	Phocomelia, limb hypoplasia, ear and cardiac anomalies	Days 21–36 post-LMP (weeks 4–5)
Cocaine	Fetal hypoxia, hypertension, growth restriction in rodents	Intrauterine growth restriction (IUGR), placental abruption, preterm labor	Throughout pregnancy
Ethanol	Microencephaly, limb, and craniofacial anomalies in rodents	Fetal alcohol syndrome: CNS dysfunction, facial anomalies, growth retardation	Throughout pregnancy, mainly in the 1st trimester
Lithium	Cardiac anomalies in rats	Ebstein's anomaly (tricuspid valve malformation)	Weeks 4–6

CNS = Central nervous system; LMP = Last menstrual period.

Table 2.
Examples of teratogenic drugs with documented effects in humans, based on animal and clinical data (adapted and modified from Gupta R.C. [23]).

of kernicterus in glucose-6-phosphate dehydrogenase (G6PD)-deficient infants [25]. Aminoglycosides, although rarely used during pregnancy, have been associated with ototoxicity and potential auditory damage in exposed infants. These effects illustrate how neonatal pharmacokinetics, particularly limited protein binding, immature enzyme systems, and underdeveloped renal filtration, can increase vulnerability to adverse outcomes [26].

In addition to direct toxicity, neonates may also present with withdrawal symptoms, a condition commonly referred to as neonatal abstinence syndrome (NAS). This syndrome is most frequently observed after prolonged in utero exposure to central nervous system (CNS) active drugs, particularly opioids (illicit substances or theoretical agents), benzodiazepines, barbiturates, and, though less consistently, selective serotonin reuptake inhibitors (SSRIs) [27–29]. Affected infants may exhibit signs such as tremors, irritability, inconsolable crying, poor feeding, vomiting, diarrhea, hypertonia, and, in severe cases, seizures. Onset typically occurs within 24–72 hours after birth, depending on the half-life of the drug and the timing of the last maternal dose. Management strategies include supportive care, rooming-in with the mother, and, when necessary, pharmacologic treatment with agents such as morphine or phenobarbital. Hospital stays for infants with NAS may be prolonged and resource-intensive, highlighting the importance of early identification and multidisciplinary care.

Beyond the immediate postnatal period, concern also exists regarding the long-term neurodevelopmental consequences of certain drug exposures during pregnancy. For example, exposure to valproic acid has been robustly linked to cognitive impairment and an increased risk of autism spectrum disorders (ASD), even in the absence of major congenital malformations. Other antiepileptic drugs may carry similar, albeit less pronounced, risks [30]. The use of SSRIs during late pregnancy has been associated in some studies with subtle neurobehavioral changes in offspring, including increased emotional reactivity, sleep disturbances, and delayed psychomotor development, although the evidence is mixed and causality remains uncertain. Similarly, the use of corticosteroids—often necessary to enhance fetal lung maturity—has raised questions about potential long-term effects on the hypothalamic–pituitary–adrenal axis and stress responses later in life [31]. Additionally, the administration of the antenatal axis and stress responsiveness in later life [32]. **Figure 2** summarizes the most important drugs/drug classes that should be avoided during pregnancy or used only when the potential benefits outweigh the risks.

Due to fears of teratogenic effects, necessary medications are often under-prescribed, deprescribed, or stopped during pregnancy—sometimes by healthcare providers and sometimes by the mothers themselves. However, such precautionary withholding of treatment can result in poorly controlled maternal conditions, such as depression, anxiety, or epilepsy, which themselves pose significant risks to both the mother and the fetus. The consequences of untreated chronic diseases may include preterm birth, fetal growth restriction, and maternal morbidity. Therefore, therapeutic decision-making in pregnancy must carefully weigh not only the

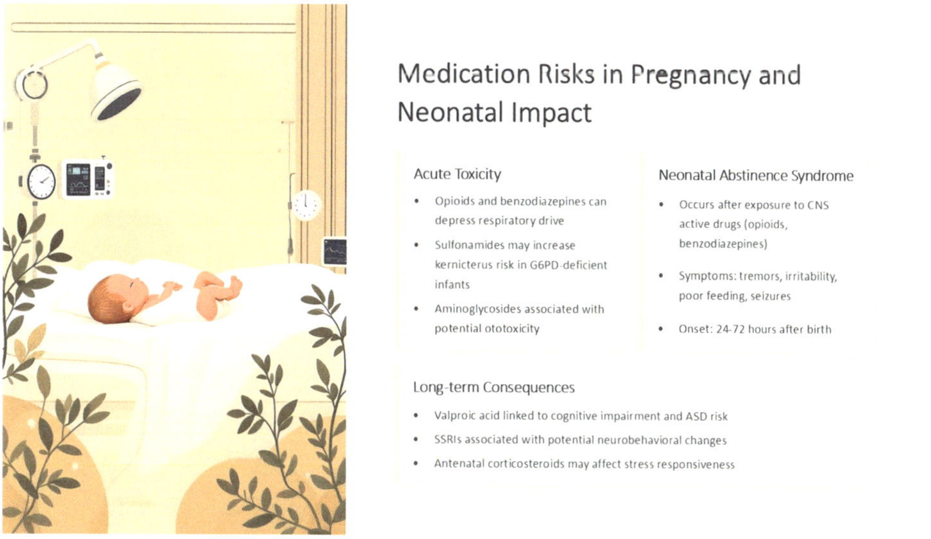

Figure 2.
Drugs and drug classes with potential neonatal risks.

theoretical teratogenic risks but also the well-documented dangers of inadequate maternal care, highlighting the need for evidence-based, individualized treatment approaches [33].

Importantly, much of the available evidence comes from observational studies, cohort data, or pregnancy registries, due to the ethical impossibility of conducting randomized controlled trials in this population. This highlights the importance of long-term follow-up of exposed children and the development of comprehensive pregnancy safety registries that can inform future guidelines and prescribing decisions.

3.3 Breastfeeding safety: Drug transfer into breast milk, accumulation, toxicity

Breastfeeding provides unparalleled nutritional, immunological, and psychological benefits to infants, contributing to optimal growth, neurodevelopment, and maternal–infant bonding. International guidelines from the World Health Organization and the American Academy of Pediatrics strongly recommend breastfeeding even when maternal pharmacotherapy is necessary, provided the medications involved are compatible with lactation [34]. Discontinuation should occur only when the risks of drug exposure clearly outweigh the benefits of breastfeeding.

Most pharmacological treatments do not require cessation of breastfeeding. Numerous studies and expert consensus now emphasize that many commonly used medications are compatible with breastfeeding and can be safely administered when selected and monitored appropriately [35, 36]. Key considerations include the drug's transfer into breast milk, its oral bioavailability to the infant, and the developmental maturity of the infant's metabolism and excretion pathways.

Despite growing evidence, misconceptions persist among healthcare professionals and the public, often leading to unnecessary cessation of breastfeeding. Observational studies indicate that both prescribers and mothers may interrupt lactation out of fear or uncertainty rather than actual risk [37, 38]. This underscores the need for better education, accessible resources, and shared decision-making strategies. Informational tools such as the Drugs and Lactation Database (LactMed®, www.ncbi.nlm.nih.gov/books/NBK501922/) and national guidelines (e.g., NICE NG194) are essential to support evidence-based choices and promote maternal autonomy.

The lack of standardized lactation-specific drug safety classifications complicates clinical decision-making. Unlike the older Food and Drug Administration (FDA) pregnancy categories, which are now replaced by the narrative-format Pregnancy and Lactation Labeling Rule (PLLR) (see paragraph 4.1), lactation safety data are often limited and derived from case reports, observational studies, or physiologically-based pharmacokinetic (PBPK) modeling [39]. These resources provide up-to-date information regarding the safety of medicinal products during pregnancy and breastfeeding according to the most recent recommendations.

Pharmacokinetic factors such as low oral bioavailability, short half-life, high protein binding, and poor lipid solubility generally limit drug transfer into breast milk. Still, certain medications, such as cytotoxic agents (i.e., methotrexate, cyclophosphamide), high-dose corticosteroids (i.e., prednisone >20 mg/day) [40], or radioisotopes (i.e., iodine-131, gallium-67) [41, 42] are contraindicated or require breastfeeding interruption [43]. In contrast, drugs like paracetamol, ibuprofen, most SSRIs, and several antihypertensives are considered compatible [35, 40]. Among antihypertensives, labetalol is noted for its low milk transfer and negligible infant exposure, making it a preferred agent during lactation [44]. Similarly, sertraline (SSRIs) is considered safe during breastfeeding [45].

Crucially, individual maternal health needs must not be overlooked. Conditions such as postpartum depression, hypertension, or posttransplant immunosuppression may necessitate ongoing therapy. In these cases, deprescription or interruption of breastfeeding can have adverse consequences for both mother and infant. Multidisciplinary care, including pharmacological counseling and maternal mental health support, facilitates safe and sustained breastfeeding [35, 46].

The safety of pharmacotherapy during lactation must be assessed within a framework that centers maternal well-being and infant protection while preserving breastfeeding whenever possible. Empowering women with accurate information and involving them in therapeutic decisions promotes both autonomy and health equity. A proactive, evidence-based approach (grounded in advocacy, individualized risk assessment, and multidisciplinary collaboration) is essential for ensuring safe and continued breastfeeding in the context of necessary medical treatment.

Finally, medications can also be used to suppress lactation: these are primarily represented by the active ingredients bromocriptine and cabergoline, which have replaced the hormonal therapies used in past decades [47]. The Australian Breastfeeding Association recommends using these medications shortly after childbirth, as their effectiveness decreases significantly after weeks or months of breastfeeding. Furthermore, stopping breastfeeding through the use of dopaminergic agonists may lead to breast engorgement or mastitis and could cause a rebound effect with the return of lactation. For these reasons, it is crucial to discuss the benefits and risks of each treatment with a healthcare professional [48]. **Table 3** summarizes drugs mentioned in the text according to their compatibility with breastfeeding, distinguishing between commonly used safe medications and those requiring caution or contraindication.

Drug/Class	Example(s)	Lactation safety	Notes
Analgesics	Paracetamol, Ibuprofen	✓ Compatible	First-line options for pain and fever; minimal transfer into breast milk
Antidepressants (SSRIs)	Sertraline	✓ Compatible	Most SSRIs have low milk levels; sertraline often preferred
Antihypertensives	Labetalol	✓ Compatible	Commonly used in postpartum hypertension
Cytotoxic agents	Methotrexate, Cyclophosphamide	× Contraindicated	High toxicity; breastfeeding should be avoided
Corticosteroids (high dose)	Prednisone (>20 mg/day)	⚠ Caution	Temporary interruption may be considered after high doses
Radioisotopes	Iodine-131 and Gallium-67	× Contraindicated	Require temporary or permanent cessation of breastfeeding
Dopaminergic agonists	Bromocriptine, Cabergoline	× Contraindicated	Used intentionally to stop breastfeeding

Table 3.
Overview of commonly used drugs during breastfeeding and drugs not allowed.

4. Drug risk classification systems

Starting from preclinical studies on animal models, anecdotal evidence, and/or observational studies, various drug classification systems have been developed that divide drugs into risk classes based on their teratogenic potential.

4.1 FDA system (legacy A, B, C, D, X, and new PLLR—Pregnancy and Lactation Labeling Rule)

The former Food and Drug Administration (FDA) pregnancy risk categories provided a system for classifying the potential harm of a drug to the fetus based on available evidence [49]. The classification considered both the quality of the data and the overall balance between potential risks and therapeutic benefits for the mother. The five categories were:

- *Category A*: Controlled studies in humans show no risk;
- *Category B*: Animal studies show no risk, or animal studies show risk but human studies do not;
- *Category C*: Animal studies show risk, and there are no adequate human studies, or there are no animal or human studies;
- *Category D*: There is evidence of risk to the human fetus, but the potential benefits of the drug in certain situations may outweigh the risks;
- *Category X*: Studies in animals or humans have demonstrated fetal abnormalities, and the risks of the drug outweigh any potential benefit.

The PLLR, currently in use, replaced the previous letter-based categorization with a more detailed narrative format. Rather than assigning a single letter grade to summarize risk, drug labeling now includes dedicated sections—"Pregnancy" and "Lactation"—that outline known risks, clinical considerations, and supporting data. This update was designed to help healthcare professionals and patients make better-informed decisions by offering clearer, more comprehensive information regarding medication use during pregnancy and breastfeeding [50].

4.2 AU TGA categories (A, B1, B2, B3, C, D, X)

In Australia, the Therapeutic Goods Administration (TGA) uses a classification system to assess the safety of medicines during pregnancy, assigning them to categories A, B1, B2, B3, C, D, and X. This system reflects the potential risk posed to the fetus, with Category A indicating the most favorable safety profile and Category X identifying drugs that are contraindicated due to known harmful effects. Primarily intended for use by healthcare professionals, this framework supports informed prescribing decisions in the context of pregnancy [51]. Below is an overview of each category within the Australian TGA pregnancy classification system:

- *Category A*: Widely used in pregnant women without any proven risk of fetal harm or malformations;

- *Category B1*: Limited human use with no observed fetal harm, and animal studies show no risk;
- *Category B2*: Limited human data with no evidence of fetal harm, and animal data are inadequate or lacking, but available findings are reassuring;
- *Category B3*: Limited human use with no observed harm; however, animal studies show signs of fetal damage;
- *Category C*: May cause harmful effects on the fetus or newborn (excluding malformations), and effects are usually reversible;
- *Category D*: Evidence or suspicion of increased risk of fetal malformations or irreversible harm, and may also have harmful pharmacological effects;
- *Category X*: High risk of permanent fetal damage and contraindicated in pregnancy or in women who may become pregnant.

4.3 Importance of individualized clinical judgment over rigid categories

Both the FDA and the Australian TGA have developed classification systems to inform the safe use of medications during pregnancy. However, they differ significantly in format and intended purpose.

The PLLR, with its narrative format, is designed to offer more comprehensive, contextualized information, including details on potential risks, benefits, and clinical considerations across three sections: Pregnancy, Lactation, and Females and Males of Reproductive Potential. The goal is to support informed, evidence-based prescribing by providing information that goes beyond an oversimplified letter grade, since a single letter often fails to capture the complexity of drug safety and could be misleading or unclear, both for healthcare professionals and for patients. By contrast, the Australian TGA system continues to use a letter-based categorization grounded primarily in the type and quality of available scientific evidence, particularly from human and animal data. Although more structured than the former FDA letters, this system is designed primarily for professional use and does not necessarily convey the full clinical context.

Ultimately, while both systems offer valuable guidance, no classification scheme can replace individualized clinical judgment. Safe prescribing during pregnancy requires a nuanced evaluation of the risk–benefit balance for both the mother and the fetus, taking into account factors such as gestational age, maternal condition, dosage, duration of therapy, and availability of safer alternatives. In many cases, withholding treatment may pose greater risks than the medication itself. For this reason, classification systems should be seen as tools to support therapeutic decisions, decisions that must always be tailored to the individual clinical scenario.

5. Epidemiology and prevalence of drug use in pregnancy and lactation

An increasing body of evidence has emerged regarding medication use in pregnancy and lactation, highlighting both the prevalence of drug exposure and the associated clinical implications.

A study conducted in New Zealand [52] analyzed prescriptions issued to pregnant women between 2005 and 2015. The analysis showed that the proportion of women exposed to at least one prescription increased from 38.5 to 67.2%, with the average number of prescribed drugs rising from 2 to 3 therapies. A subsequent analysis [53] evaluated the prescription of drugs potentially harmful to the fetus, specifically those classified as Category D and X according to the Australian pregnancy risk categorization system (https://www.tga.gov.au/prescribing-medicines-pregnancy-database). Drugs in Category D were dispensed during 4.3% of pregnancies, while those in Category X were dispensed during 0.058%. These drugs were more frequently prescribed before conception, with prescription rates decreasing as pregnancy progressed. Another study conducted in the Netherlands [54] found that drug use occurred in 73% of the pregnancies analyzed, and 34% of these involved potentially harmful medications. The use of such treatments was associated with chronic disease management, particularly diabetes, thyroid disorders, migraine, epilepsy, psychiatric conditions, depression, and asthma. A pharmacoepidemiological study carried out in Belgium [55] using administrative database records from 2003 to 2017 showed an increase in the number of medications to which pregnant women were exposed, with a rise in average drug count from 2 to 3. The prevalence of women exposed to pharmacological treatments increased from 82% to 89%. The most frequently prescribed drugs were progesterone, paracetamol, and amoxicillin.

Harvard and colleagues [56] assessed medication use in pregnant women in New South Wales (Australia) between 2006 and 2012. Medications more likely to be prescribed to pregnant women than to nonpregnant women included antacids, ranitidine, sodium alginate combined with calcium carbonate and bicarbonate, ondansetron, insulin and insulin analogues, antithrombotic and antiplatelet agents (enoxaparin, dalteparin, and acetylsalicylic acid), iron preparations, vitamin B12 and folic acid, methyldopa, hydralazine, nifedipine, clotrimazole, antibiotics and antivirals (e.g., ampicillin, amoxicillin, clindamycin, acyclovir), budesonide, and ipratropium.

A cross-sectional study conducted in Europe, North and South America, and Australia examined patterns and factors associated with medication use, the most commonly used pharmacological classes, and their indications [57]. Data collected *via* questionnaire from a sample of over 9000 pregnant women or women who had given birth in the previous year showed that 81.2% had used at least one prescription or over-the-counter (OTC) medication. The highest prevalence of drug use was observed in the Netherlands (95.1%), Iceland (93%), and Finland (92.3%). According to the Anatomical Therapeutic Chemical (ATC) classification, the most frequently reported classes were drugs acting on the nervous system, analgesics (ATC class N01*, largely represented by paracetamol), psycholeptics (ATC class N05*), and psychoanaleptics (ATC class N06*); drugs for the gastrointestinal tract—mainly antacids (ATC class A02*) and laxatives (ATC class A06*); drugs for the respiratory system, especially nasal preparations (ATC class R01*) and antihistamines (ATC class R06*); and systemic antibiotics (ATC class J01*). The main indications for acute or short-term treatment included headache, heartburn, pain, nausea, and urinary tract infections. Chronic or long-term treatments were more common in North America, Northern Europe, and Australia compared to Western Europe. Factors most associated with such treatments included older maternal age, unemployment, and unplanned pregnancy.

A follow-up analysis of this study [58] focused solely on Italian participants and found that 61.4% of the sample used medication for acute conditions, 12.4%

Study/Country	Period	Key findings	Notes/Risk categories
New Zealand [47]	2005–2015	Drug exposure increased from 38.5% to 67.2%; the average number of drugs per pregnancy increased from 2 to 3.	—
New Zealand [48]	2005–2015	Category D drugs in 4.3% of pregnancies; Category X in 0.058%. Prescriptions decreased as pregnancy progressed.	Australian risk categorization system (Categories D and X).
Netherlands [49]	1999–2017	Drug use in 73% of pregnancies; 34% included potentially harmful drugs.	Associated with chronic conditions (e.g., diabetes, epilepsy, psychiatric disorders).
Belgium [50]	2003–2017	Drug exposure increased from 2 to 3 medications; prevalence rose from 82% to 89%.	Most prescribed: progesterone, paracetamol, amoxicillin.
Australia (NSW) [51]	2006–2012	More likely prescribed in pregnancy: antacids, ondansetron, insulin analogs, antithrombotics, iron, folic acid, antihypertensives, antibiotics.	Compared to nonpregnant women.
Multicontinental study [52]	2011–2012	81.2% of women used ≥1 medication (Rx or OTC); higher prevalence in NL (95.1%), IS (93%), FI (92.3%).	Most used drug classes: analgesics (ATC N01*), GI drugs (A02*, A06*), respiratory meds (R01*, R06*), antibiotics (J01*).
Italy (subset) [53]	2011–2012	Acute drug use: 61.4%; chronic: 12.4%; both: 8.8%. High use of paracetamol with antacids and/or antibiotics.	Notable use of benzodiazepines and antidepressants, especially in the 1st trimester.

Category D/X drugs = Medications known or suspected to harm the fetus (see the TGA Australia database).
ATC = Anatomical Therapeutic Chemical classification system; OTC = Over-the-counter medication.

Table 4.
Overview of drug use in pregnancy across different countries and study settings.

for chronic diseases, and 8.8% for both types of treatment. In addition to pain and urinary tract infections, an important indication for drug use was the management of disorders in women with a history of alcohol abuse prior to pregnancy. The most common drug combinations were paracetamol and antacids (13.3%), paracetamol and antibiotics (11.7%), paracetamol and prokinetics (6.5%), and antacids with antibiotics (4.2%). Notably, the use of benzodiazepines and antidepressants was higher in the first trimester compared to later stages of pregnancy.

Table 4 summarizes major findings from international studies on medication use in pregnancy, with emphasis on prescription trends, fetal risk categories, and associated maternal conditions.

6. Medications and natural products: Key examples

6.1 Antidepressants

The use of selective serotonin reuptake inhibitors (SSRIs) during pregnancy is a topic of considerable clinical interest, particularly concerning their association with various neonatal and maternal outcomes. Extensive literature has explored the implications of SSRI exposure on NAS, congenital malformations, preterm birth, and other perinatal outcomes.

Exposure to SSRIs, especially in the third trimester, has been linked to an increased incidence of NAS, also referred to as poor neonatal adaptation syndrome (PNAS). This condition is characterized by symptoms such as irritability, tremors, respiratory difficulties, feeding problems, muscle tone abnormalities, and sleep disturbances. Less frequently, lethargy, weak cry, hypoglycemia, and seizures may occur. Approximately 25–30% of neonates exposed to SSRIs exhibit signs of NAS [59]. Symptoms typically emerge within the first 48 hours but can be delayed to days 5–7 and persist for 2–4 weeks [60]. The 2024 UK neonatal guidelines recommend hospital birth and 48-hour observation for infants with third-trimester SSRI exposure. Informed refusal is permitted and not classified as a safeguarding concern.

Meta-analyses have suggested a modest increase in the risk of major congenital malformations, particularly cardiac defects, with first-trimester SSRI exposure (Relative Risk, RR ~1.11–1.24), especially with fluoxetine, paroxetine, and sertraline [61]. Specifically, fluoxetine has been associated with a 30–40% increase in the risk of ventricular septal defects [62]. However, the 2024 UK guideline notes that overall, there is no consistent association with congenital abnormalities, though a small excess risk of cardiac anomalies cannot be ruled out. A small but measurable increase in Persistent Pulmonary Hypertension of the Newborn (PPHN) has been observed following late gestational SSRI exposure. Estimates suggest that 286–351 pregnancies exposed in the third trimester are needed to result in one additional case [63]. Early detection improves outcomes. The Royal Cornwall Hospitals Trust (RCHT) guideline advises discussing PPHN risks during antenatal counseling [59].

Multiple meta-analyses and large cohort studies indicate that SSRI use is associated with an increased risk of preterm birth [Odds Ratio (OR) 1.5–1.9] and low birth weight (OR 1.5–1.7), particularly when exposure occurs after the first trimester [59–67] (**Table 5**). Notably, no significant association has been found between SSRI use and small for gestational age (SGA) [64].

While earlier studies raised concern about a potential increase in miscarriage risk, more recent evidence does not confirm a significant association. In contrast, SSRIs are associated with slightly elevated risks of preeclampsia and postpartum hemorrhage [61, 65].

The relationship between prenatal SSRI exposure and neurodevelopmental disorders, including ASD and attention-deficit/hyperactivity disorder (ADHD), remains controversial. Systematic reviews have failed to establish a consistent causal link, and many studies suggest that maternal psychiatric illness itself may account for much of the observed association [58, 65].

Outcome	Odds Ratio (OR)	Exposure timing	Association
Preterm birth	1.5–1.9	Especially after the 1st trimester	Significant
Low birth weight	1.5–1.7	Especially after the 1st trimester	Significant
SGA	Not significant	Any	None

SGA = Small for gestation age.

Table 5.
Outcomes associated with the use of SSRIs.

In clinical practice, sertraline is frequently preferred during pregnancy and breastfeeding due to lower placental transfer and reduced breast milk excretion [59]. Fluoxetine, in contrast, has a long half-life and is found in higher concentrations in breast milk, which may increase the risk of PNAS and PPHN. Despite these differences, both drugs are considered acceptable options when the benefits outweigh potential risks. Some data suggest a 29–42% relative increase in cardiac anomalies with sertraline [68], though the absolute risk remains low.

6.2 Antiepileptics

The use of antiepileptic drugs (AEDs) during pregnancy requires a careful balance between maintaining maternal seizure control and minimizing risks to the developing fetus. While untreated epilepsy can pose significant dangers, including maternal injury and hypoxic events for the fetus, certain AEDs carry substantial teratogenic and neurodevelopmental risks. Among all AEDs, valproate is associated with the highest risk of major congenital malformations (MCMs), with estimates ranging from 9 to 10% or higher depending on dose and timing of exposure. Malformations include neural tube defects, facial dysmorphism, cardiac anomalies, and urogenital malformations [66–71]. Topiramate and phenobarbital also pose significant risks, including increased rates of oral clefts (topiramate) and cardiac defects or growth restriction (phenobarbital), although less pronounced than valproate [67, 68, 72]. Conversely, lamotrigine and levetiracetam are associated with a low risk of MCMs, comparable to background population rates (2–3.5%), and are generally considered safer options for monotherapy [66–69, 71]. Carbamazepine has an intermediate risk, particularly dose-dependent, for neural tube defects and craniofacial anomalies [69]. Oxcarbazepine, a structural analogue, appears safer, though data remain limited and further studies are needed [71].

In addition to structural malformations, in utero exposure to AEDs has been associated with neurodevelopmental disorders, including cognitive delay, ASD, and ADHD. Valproate remains the most concerning agent, with strong evidence linking prenatal exposure to lower IQ scores, ASD, and impaired language development [69–71, 73]. Some data also indicate neurodevelopmental risks with phenobarbital, carbamazepine, and possibly topiramate, though the evidence is less consistent. Lamotrigine and levetiracetam are associated with lower risks of developmental delay, although levetiracetam has been linked in some studies to increased rates of ADHD and anxiety symptoms [69]. Oxcarbazepine has shown a possible correlation with ASD, but current evidence remains insufficient for definitive conclusions [71, 73].

Pharmacokinetic changes during pregnancy, including increased renal clearance, altered plasma protein binding, and induced hepatic metabolism, can lead to reduced serum levels of several AEDs. In particular, lamotrigine clearance increases significantly from the first trimester onward, often requiring dose adjustments to maintain therapeutic levels [74–76]. Therapeutic drug monitoring (TDM) is recommended for lamotrigine, levetiracetam, and oxcarbazepine throughout pregnancy to avoid both subtherapeutic exposure and toxicity [71, 76]. The results of these studies are summarized in **Table 6**.

High-dose folic acid supplementation ($\geq$4 mg/day) is advised for all women taking AEDs, especially those on valproate or carbamazepine, to mitigate the risk of neural tube defects. However, the optimal dose for neuroprotection is still under investigation [69, 71]. Given the heterogeneity of AED safety profiles, individualized treatment planning is essential. Where clinically appropriate, lamotrigine or levetiracetam

AED	MCM risk	Neurodevelopmental risk	Notes
Valproate	High (≥10%)	High (ASD, IQ↓, psychomotor delay)	Avoid if possible; strongly dose-dependent
Phenobarbital	Moderate–High	Moderate	Cognitive impact documented
Topiramate	Moderate	Some risk (cleft lip, uncertain NDD)	Avoid if alternatives exist
Lamotrigine	Low	Low	Preferred; requires TDM
Levetiracetam	Low	ADHD/anxiety (some evidence)	Preferred; monitor during pregnancy
Carbamazepine	Moderate	Moderate; dose-related	Avoid high doses
Oxcarbazepine	Low–Moderate	Possible autism risk	Limited data; generally well-tolerated

ADHD = Attention-deficit/hyperactivity disorder; AED = Antiepileptic drug; ASD = Autism spectrum disorder; MCM = Major congenital malformations; TDM = Therapeutic drug monitoring.

Table 6.
AEDs and pregnancy safety (adapted from Andrade et al. [66], and Nucera et al. [71]).

should be considered as first-line options during pregnancy. Avoidance of valproate, particularly during the first trimester, is strongly recommended. Close monitoring of serum drug levels and maternal-fetal well-being throughout gestation is critical to optimize outcomes.

6.3 Antibiotics

Antibiotics are among the most frequently prescribed medications during pregnancy, primarily to treat urinary tract infections, bacterial vaginosis, and other infections that, if left untreated, may jeopardize maternal and fetal health. The safety profile of each antibiotic class must be carefully evaluated, as certain agents are considered safe and effective, while others may pose risks of teratogenicity, fetotoxicity, or long-term developmental effects. Most beta-lactam antibiotics, including penicillins and cephalosporins, are generally considered safe for use in all trimesters, with substantial evidence from both human and animal studies supporting their use. Similarly, other antibiotics such as clindamycin, metronidazole, and fosfomycin also exhibit favorable safety profiles. Nitrofurantoin is typically safe during early and mid-pregnancy, but its use is discouraged near term due to the risk of hemolytic anemia in neonates with glucose-6-phosphate dehydrogenase (G6PD) deficiency [77, 78]. In contrast, some antibiotics are associated with significant fetal risk and are best avoided. Tetracyclines, for instance, can impair fetal bone growth and cause permanent tooth discoloration, especially with second and third trimester exposure [79]. Fluoroquinolones have shown the potential to damage fetal cartilage in animal models and are generally contraindicated in pregnancy [77]. Trimethoprim-sulfamethoxazole (TMP-SMX), although sometimes necessary, has been linked to neural tube defects and miscarriage when used during early gestation, due to its folate-antagonist properties [80, 81]. Macrolides show mixed safety data: while some studies suggest acceptable profiles, others raise concerns about possible associations with miscarriage or adverse reproductive outcomes, especially when used preconceptionally [81].

Antibiotic exposure during pregnancy also raises concerns beyond teratogenicity. Disruption of maternal and fetal microbiota is a growing area of research, with evidence indicating that prenatal antibiotic use may affect neonatal immune system development and increase susceptibility to asthma, allergies, and metabolic diseases later in life [82, 83]. Broad-spectrum agents may exert more profound microbiome shifts, underscoring the importance of antibiotic stewardship in perinatal care [84, 85].

The benefits of treating infections during pregnancy generally outweigh potential risks, particularly in cases of urinary tract infections, which are common and can lead to serious complications if untreated. Clinical guidelines support the use of appropriately selected antibiotics in these contexts, with amoxicillin, nitrofurantoin, and cephalosporins remaining first-line options in many protocols [86, 87]. Lastly, attention must be paid to preconception antibiotic exposure, as emerging data suggest that certain antibiotics, including macrolides and sulfonamides, may negatively affect fertility and early pregnancy outcomes when administered during the periconceptional period [81].

In summary, the rational use of antibiotics in pregnancy should follow a risk–benefit analysis that weighs the necessity of infection control against the known or suspected risks of each compound. While many antibiotics have proven safety records, others require caution or should be avoided altogether. Prescribers must remain up-to-date with evolving safety data and practice evidence-based selection and dosing to safeguard both maternal and fetal health.

6.4 Analgesics and anti-inflammatory agents

Pain management during pregnancy presents a unique challenge, requiring a careful balance between maternal comfort and fetal safety. Among the most commonly used medications in this context are paracetamol (acetaminophen), nonsteroidal anti-inflammatory drugs (NSAIDs), and opioids. Each class carries distinct safety profiles depending on the timing, dosage, and duration of use.

Paracetamol (acetaminophen) is widely regarded as the safest analgesic during all trimesters of pregnancy and is considered first-line treatment for mild to moderate pain or fever. It has a long history of use and a favorable safety profile when used at recommended doses. Nevertheless, emerging evidence has raised concerns regarding potential long-term neurodevelopmental effects, such as behavioral or attention disorders, in children exposed in utero, although causality remains unconfirmed, and confounding factors (e.g., maternal health) may play a substantial role [88, 89].

NSAIDs (e.g., ibuprofen, naproxen, and diclofenac) pose more complex risks. While occasionally used in the first and early second trimester, evidence links NSAIDs to an increased risk of spontaneous miscarriage and specific congenital anomalies, including orofacial clefts [90]. The use of NSAIDs after 20 weeks of gestation is particularly concerning due to the risk of fetal renal dysfunction, oligohydramnios, and premature closure of the ductus arteriosus, a vital fetal blood vessel. These risks escalate in the third trimester, and guidelines therefore advise avoiding NSAIDs during this period altogether [91–93]. Low-dose aspirin may be used with clear clinical indications, such as the prevention of preeclampsia in high-risk pregnancies. However, routine or high-dose use in later pregnancy is discouraged due to risks of fetal bleeding, ductal closure, and impaired labor [94, 95].

Opioids may be necessary in cases of severe or refractory pain, such as that associated with trauma or major surgical procedures. When used briefly and under supervision, they can be considered safe, especially in early pregnancy. However, chronic or late-pregnancy exposure is associated with NAS. Respiratory depression may also occur immediately after birth, particularly if opioids were administered intrapartum [96].

Table 7 summarizes the evidence regarding the use of analgesics and anti-inflammatory drugs during pregnancy.

In conclusion, while pharmacologic pain relief is often necessary during pregnancy, it must be carefully individualized. Paracetamol (acetaminophen) remains the safest first-line option, while NSAIDs and opioids require more nuanced consideration of timing, indication, and potential fetal outcomes. A risk–benefit approach, integrated with patient counseling and pharmacovigilance, is essential to ensure safe and effective maternal care.

6.5 Use of herbal and natural products during pregnancy

The use of herbal and natural products during pregnancy is common across diverse cultures and socioeconomic groups, largely driven by the belief that "natural" means "safe." However, this assumption is not supported by solid scientific evidence. The safety of most herbal products in pregnancy remains poorly defined, with variability in composition, pharmacological effects, and the ability of active compounds to cross the placenta. Despite their widespread use, these substances are often understudied in pregnant populations, and clinical pharmacology has traditionally focused on conventional drugs. In this context, phytovigilance and observational research are essential to better understand their safety profiles. Herbal products, though perceived as benign, can interact with maternal physiology, other medications, and fetal development, and may range from harmless to potentially harmful [97].

Among the most frequently used herbal products in pregnancy, ginger (*Zingiber officinale*) is the most extensively studied. When consumed at doses below 1000 mg/day, it has demonstrated efficacy in reducing nausea and vomiting during early pregnancy, with no significant increase in adverse outcomes for mother or fetus. However, high doses may pose gastrointestinal or anticoagulant risks, especially if used concomitantly with other substances with similar profiles [98]. Conversely, other widely used herbs lack sufficient safety data or have demonstrated concerning effects. *St. John's Wort* (*Hypericum perforatum*), used to treat depressive symptoms, has been associated with teratogenic and pharmacokinetic risks and is generally not recommended during pregnancy [99, 100]. *Ginseng*, *Ginkgo biloba*, and *Aloe vera* have

Drug class	Safe in early pregnancy	Safe in late pregnancy	Main risks in late pregnancy
Paracetamol	Yes	Yes	Minimal if used appropriately
NSAIDs	With caution	No	Ductus arteriosus closure, renal impairment, oligohydramnios
Aspirin (low-dose)	Yes, if indicated	No	Fetal bleeding, ductal closure
Opioids	Short-term use only	Caution	NAS, respiratory depression

ADHD = Attention-deficit/hyperactivity disorder; AED = Antiepileptic drug; ASD = Autism spectrum disorder; MCM = Major congenital malformations; TDM = Therapeutic drug monitoring.

Table 7.
Safety considerations for common analgesics and anti-inflammatory drugs during pregnancy (modified from Paech and Bloor, Ref. [94], Reis and Källén, Ref. [95], and Antonucci et al., Ref. [91]).

been flagged for potential reproductive toxicity or abortifacient activity in animal studies and human case reports, warranting caution or contraindication [101]. Other herbs, such as *Echinacea* [102] and *Evening Primrose Oil*, are commonly consumed but supported by inconsistent and insufficient evidence [103]. Some observational data suggest they may be safe in the short term, but their long-term fetal impact remains unclear. Chinese herbal medicines (CHMs) are also widely used, especially in Asian populations [104]. While some clinical and preclinical studies suggest benefits in conditions such as threatened miscarriage, concerns persist regarding quality control, standardization, and safety during early gestation. For example, hyperforin from *Hypericum* and valerenic acid from *Valeriana* species show variable transplacental passage in *ex vivo* studies, raising questions about fetal exposure levels [99].

Data from the herbal supplements in breastfeeding invesTigation (HaBIT) studies in Italy indicate that over half of breastfeeding women reported using complementary and alternative medicines (CAMs), with herbal products among the most common. Women with a history of pregnancy loss were more likely to use herbal remedies, possibly reflecting a stronger preference for perceived "safer" self-care strategies. Midwives were the main source of advice, highlighting the role of informal guidance outside traditional medical oversight. Notably, many women believed herbal products to be safer than conventional drugs, despite acknowledging limited scientific evidence. Misclassification, poor risk awareness, and reported side effects were also frequent [105, 106]. A study among Italian herbalists revealed a low perceived risk associated with most commonly sold medicinal plants, including *Echinacea*, *Aloe vera*, and *Allium sativum*, despite expert panels attributing higher risk scores to several of these substances. This discrepancy highlights a broader problem: public and commercial actors often underestimate the pharmacological activity, and therefore the potential harm, of "natural" products [107].

From a clinical toxicology standpoint, pregnant women remain "therapeutic orphans," with both conventional and alternative therapies lacking comprehensive safety data [97]. The spontaneous and unmonitored use of herbal remedies, coupled with underreporting to healthcare providers, increases the risk of drug–herb interactions, unanticipated side effects, and mismanagement of symptoms that would benefit from evidence-based treatment. For example, data from the PHYTO.VIG.GEST study reveals that while some products are well-tolerated and have reassuring safety records during pregnancy, herbal substances lack similar robust monitoring frameworks [108]. Therefore, risk minimization strategies must include not only pharmacovigilance but also structured education of both patients and healthcare providers.

Self-medication, misinformation, and the cultural valorization of "naturalness" compound the risk of inappropriate use. Comprehensive risk–benefit evaluation, proactive counseling during prenatal care, and increased research investment are needed to ensure maternal-fetal safety in an era of widespread CAM use.

7. Rational prescribing and deprescribing strategies

Rational prescribing during pregnancy requires a careful and individualized risk–benefit assessment, balancing the therapeutic advantages for the mother against potential risks for the fetus. This evaluation must be grounded in a clearly defined clinical indication and should aim to use the minimal effective dose for the shortest necessary duration [109, 110]. Given the heightened sensitivity of fetal development, particularly during organogenesis, minimizing the duration of pharmacological exposure is critical to reducing the risk of teratogenic effects [111, 112]. Prescribers must remain informed of current clinical guidelines and periodically re-evaluate the ongoing need for treatment, especially as pregnancy progresses and physiological parameters shift. Such ongoing assessment helps prevent unnecessary polypharmacy and ensures that each pharmacological intervention remains clinically justified [113]. Ultimately, prescribing strategies must be dynamic and responsive to the evolving maternal condition. The substantial physiological changes that occur during pregnancy further underscore the importance of individualized, evidence-informed treatment decisions [114].

7.1 Deprescribing: What to stop, when, and how to monitor

Deprescribing strategies during pregnancy focus not only on identifying medications to discontinue but also on establishing appropriate timelines and monitoring protocols. The practice of deprescribing involves careful evaluation of the necessity of each medication as pregnancy progresses, emphasizing the cessation of nonessential treatments [115, 116]. For instance, medication contraindications that may arise as gestation advances necessitate re-evaluation, ensuring that any remaining pharmaceutical interventions align with current clinical guidelines [117]. Healthcare providers should monitor patients closely following deprescribing to observe for any resurgence of symptoms that may necessitate alternative interventions, which can occur particularly in cases of chronic illnesses such as asthma or autoimmune conditions [118, 119]. Successful monitoring can be facilitated through regular follow-up visits, where practitioners assess maternal and fetal well-being rigorously [120]. For medications that pose greater risks during certain trimesters, timely communication is critical. Studies have demonstrated that decisions to taper or discontinue medications should coincide with emerging evidence of fetal development timelines related to medication safety [121, 122]. Additionally, integrating registries and systematic databases can enhance monitoring and reporting mechanisms, facilitating ongoing assessment of maternal and fetal outcomes post-deprescribing [123].

7.2 Patient involvement in decision-making (shared decision-making model)

Involving patients in the shared decision-making process is vital for the successful management of medication safety during pregnancy. Research highlights that shared decision-making enhances patient knowledge and empowers women to take an active role in their own healthcare [56, 124]. The complexities surrounding medication safety in pregnancy—and the often overwhelming information available—underscore the importance of tailored patient education initiatives [125]. Providing comprehensive counseling can mitigate anxiety related to medication use, allowing for informed decisions about treatment options based on individual circumstances [126].

Furthermore, collaboration between healthcare providers and patients is essential to address the gaps in knowledge regarding medication use during pregnancy. Evidence suggests that many women are unaware of the implications of specific medications on pregnancy outcomes, reinforcing the need for ongoing dialogue about medication appropriateness [111]. Integrating feedback from patients concerning their experiences and preferences can refine treatment plans and adhere to shared decision-making principles, thereby enhancing overall treatment satisfaction [123, 127]. This approach leads to a better understanding of the patient's unique health profile as well as their mental and emotional well-being throughout pregnancy.

8. Pharmacovigilance and post-marketing surveillance: Okay, but...

Pharmacovigilance plays a crucial role in enhancing medication safety during pregnancy by monitoring adverse events associated with drug use and compiling data from a range of sources, including pregnancy registries and clinical databases [116, 123, 128]. The importance of meticulous adverse event reporting cannot be understated; it facilitates the identification of potential risks and informs clinical guidelines regarding medication use in pregnancy [129–131]. Regular updates about medications, informed by reports of adverse outcomes, allow practitioners to make evidence-based decisions that prioritize both maternal and fetal health. Pregnancy registries serve as invaluable tools in this context, collecting data on pregnant individuals exposed to specific medications and tracking outcomes [119, 123]. The systematic compilation of this data enables researchers to evaluate the safety profiles of various drugs within diverse populations, thereby addressing gaps in knowledge regarding medication use during pregnancy. These registries can help dispel myths related to drug safety and catalyze pivotal changes in prescribing practices when significant risks are identified [111].

The role of safety databases and clinical guidelines, such as LactMed and e-lactancia, is paramount, particularly in providing healthcare professionals and patients with evidence-based resources [121]. These databases aggregate existing clinical data, making it accessible for practitioners, which can lead to increased awareness and concerted efforts in mitigating risks associated with medication choices during pregnancy. Moreover, the application of such guidelines assists in harmonizing care across different healthcare settings, ensuring that all practitioners adhere to best practices [117]. Successful pharmacovigilance efforts necessitate not only data collection but also collaboration among various stakeholders, including healthcare providers, public health agencies, and patients. Engaging in dialogue about potential concerns and emerging evidence can cultivate a culture of safety within the healthcare ecosystem [109, 125]. Continuous advancements in technology and data analytics further augment these efforts, allowing for real-time monitoring of medication safety alongside developments in treatment protocols [123].

The dynamics of medication safety in pregnancy are multifaceted, encompassing strategies for rational prescribing and deprescribing, active patient involvement in clinical decision-making, and robust pharmacovigilance infrastructures. By creating an ecosystem that prioritizes both maternal and fetal safety, through informed, evidence-based practices and stakeholder collaboration, it is possible to navigate the complex landscape of pharmacotherapy during pregnancy more effectively. Continued research and adherence to safety guidelines will be paramount in ensuring that healthcare providers can offer optimized and safe medication choices for pregnant patients.

9. Practical recommendations and tools for clinicians

Prescribing medications during pregnancy presents a unique clinical challenge. **Figure 3** summarizes recommendations regarding the most commonly prescribed drug classes during pregnancy. Physiological changes, limited high-quality evidence, and ethical constraints on clinical trials all contribute to uncertainty. This reinforces the need for cautious, evidence-based, and patient-centered decision-making.

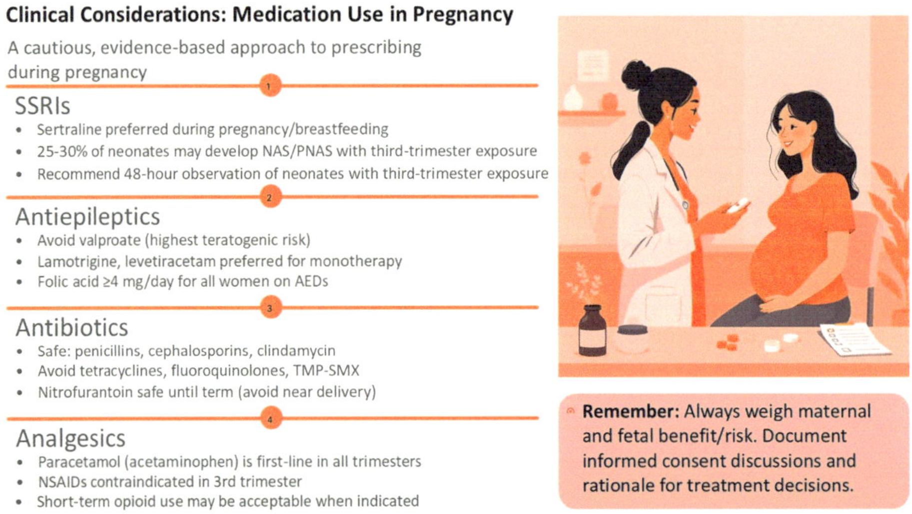

Figure 3.
Recommendations for commonly prescribed medications during pregnancy.

The following recommendations synthesize the key principles discussed throughout the chapter and aim to provide a practical guide for clinicians involved in maternal care.

- *Assess necessity carefully*: Begin by evaluating whether pharmacological treatment is truly necessary. Avoid unnecessary medications, but do not delay or withhold essential therapies, as untreated maternal conditions can pose serious risks to both mother and fetus.

- *Prioritize safety and efficacy*: Choose drugs with the most robust evidence of safety in pregnancy, preferably supported by human data, and select agents with a favorable balance between maternal benefit and fetal risk.

- *Use the minimum effective dose*: Always prescribe the lowest effective dose for the shortest duration needed, guided by clinical response and disease severity.

- *Limit polypharmacy*: Minimize the number of concurrent medications and reassess the need for ongoing treatments regularly. Adjust plans according to the clinical evolution of both pregnancy and disease.

- *Engage in multidisciplinary collaboration*: In complex cases, seek input from obstetricians, clinical pharmacologists, and disease-specific specialists, particularly when dealing with chronic conditions, polytherapy, or off-label drug use.

- *Utilize evidence-based resources*: Consult up-to-date and reliable information sources—such as published guidelines, drug safety databases, teratology information services, and pharmacovigilance networks—before prescribing.

- *Document and communicate clearly*: Provide detailed documentation of the decision-making process and ensure shared decision-making with the patient. Discuss expected benefits, potential risks, and therapeutic alternatives.

- *Incorporate pharmacovigilance and deprescribing strategies*: Consider the evolving nature of pregnancy and use long-term follow-up and reporting tools to monitor adverse outcomes and reduce unnecessary exposure when appropriate.

Ultimately, promoting safer pharmacological care in pregnancy requires not only adherence to guidelines but also individualized judgment, multidisciplinary collaboration, and transparent communication with patients. Empowering clinicians with practical tools and up-to-date evidence can help achieve the delicate balance between maternal well-being and fetal protection.

10. Conclusions

Ensuring the safe and appropriate use of medications during pregnancy and lactation is a complex yet essential component of maternal and perinatal care. Physiological changes throughout gestation significantly affect the pharmacokinetics and pharmacodynamics of many drugs, altering their absorption, distribution, metabolism, and excretion. These changes, coupled with the ethical and methodological challenges of conducting clinical trials in pregnant populations, contribute to significant gaps in evidence and uncertainty in clinical decision-making.

While only a limited number of drugs are confirmed as human teratogens, the potential for harm—ranging from congenital malformations to neonatal toxicity and long-term developmental effects—necessitates careful benefit–risk assessment for every pharmacological intervention. Timing of exposure is critical, with the embryonic period representing the highest susceptibility to structural anomalies and the fetal period more closely associated with functional impairments and growth disturbances. In addition, late-pregnancy exposure may lead to acute neonatal toxicity or withdrawal syndromes due to immature metabolic and excretory systems.

Prescribing/deprescribing decisions should prioritize maternal health while minimizing fetal risk, always considering the lowest effective dose, the shortest necessary duration, and the availability of safer alternatives. Polypharmacy should be avoided when possible, and treatment plans should be regularly reassessed in light of gestational age and evolving clinical needs. Pharmacovigilance systems and pregnancy registries are essential tools for monitoring outcomes and improving drug safety profiles.

The use of rigid risk classification systems is insufficient to guide prescribing in such a complex context. Instead, therapeutic choices must rely on updated, evidence-based sources and be informed by clinical judgment, multidisciplinary collaboration, and transparent communication with patients. In many cases, the risks of untreated maternal disease may outweigh those of pharmacological treatment. Moreover, integrating quantitative evidence with a qualitative understanding of maternal experiences and preferences enhances the safety, effectiveness, and acceptability of perinatal pharmacotherapy. A balanced, respectful, and patient-centered prescribing practice contributes significantly to the health and well-being of both mother and child.

Conflict of interest

Authors have no conflict of interest to disclose.

Appendices and nomenclature

Abbreviations

ACE	angiotensin-converting enzyme
ADHD	attention-deficit/hyperactivity disorder
AOG	age of gestation
ASD	autism spectrum disorder
ATC	anatomical therapeutic chemical classification
AU TGA	Australian Therapeutic Goods Administration
CAM	complementary and alternative medicine
CNS	central nervous system
FDA	Food and Drug Administration
GFR	glomerular filtration rate
NAS	neonatal abstinence syndrome
NICE	National Institute for Health and Care Excellence
NO	nitric oxide
OR	odds ratio
OTC	over-the-counter
PBPK	physiologically-based pharmacokinetic
PLLR	pregnancy and lactation labeling rule
PPHN	persistent pulmonary hypertension of the newborn
RR	relative risk
SGA	small for gestational age
SMX	sulfamethoxazole
SSRIs	Selective Serotonin Reuptake Inhibitor(s)
TDM	therapeutic drug monitoring
TMP	trimethoprim
WHO	World Health Organization

Nomenclature

Deprescribing	The process of tapering or stopping medications that may no longer be beneficial or may be harmful.
Embryotoxicity	Harmful effects on the embryo during early stages of development.
Evidence-based prescribing	Medication decisions based on clinical research and individual patient needs.
Fetotoxicity	Toxic effects of a substance on the developing fetus.
Herbal medicine	The use of plant-based preparations for therapeutic purposes.
Neonatal adaptation	Physiological adjustments in a newborn transitioning from intrauterine to extrauterine life.
PBPK model	Physiologically-Based Pharmacokinetic model used to predict drug behavior in special populations.
Perinatal pharmacology	The study of drug use during pregnancy, birth, and the immediate postnatal period.
Pharmacodynamics	Study of the physiological effects of drugs and their mechanisms of action.

Pharmacokinetics	Study of how drugs are absorbed, distributed, metabolized, and excreted.
Physiological changes in pregnancy	Anatomical and metabolic changes affecting drug disposition during pregnancy.
Phytovigilance	Monitoring the safety of herbal medicines and plant-based products.
Placental transfer	The movement of substances across the placenta from maternal to fetal circulation.
Polypharmacy	The use of multiple medications by a patient, often common in complex or chronic conditions.
Post-marketing surveillance	Monitoring the safety of a drug after it has been released on the market (usually identified with pharmacovigilance).
Pregnancy risk categorization	Systems used to classify medication risk during pregnancy (e.g., FDA PLLR, AU TGA).
Risk–benefit ratio	The balance between the benefits of a treatment and its potential risks.
Teratogen	An agent that can disturb the development of the embryo or fetus.

Author details

Giada Crescioli, Costanza Cacini, Roberto Bonaiuti and Alfredo Vannacci*
Department of Neurosciences, Psychology, Drug Research and Child Health, Section of Pharmacology and Toxicology, University of Florence, Florence, Italy

*Address all correspondence to: alfredo.vannacci@unifi.it

References

[1] Maternal Health. Available from: https://www.who.int/health-topics/maternal-health [Accessed: August 1, 2025]

[2] Quinney SK, Gullapelli R, Haas DM. Translational systems pharmacology studies in pregnant women. CPT: Pharmacometrics & Systems Pharmacology. 2018;7:69-81. DOI: 10.1002/psp4.12269

[3] Ayad M, Costantine MM. Epidemiology of medications use in pregnancy. Seminars in Perinatology. 2015;**39**:508-511. DOI: 10.1053/j.semperi.2015.08.002

[4] McKiever M, Frey H, Costantine MM. Challenges in conducting clinical research studies in pregnant women. Journal of Pharmacokinetics and Pharmacodynamics. 2020;**47**:287-293. DOI: 10.1007/s10928-020-09687-z

[5] Riley LE, Cahill AG, Beigi R, et al. Improving safe and effective use of drugs in pregnancy and lactation: Workshop summary. American Journal of Perinatology. 2017;**34**:826-832. DOI: 10.1055/s-0037-1598070

[6] Kazma JM, van den Anker J, Allegaert K, et al. Anatomical and physiological alterations of pregnancy. Journal of Pharmacokinetics and Pharmacodynamics. 2020;**47**:271-285. DOI: 10.1007/s10928-020-09677-1

[7] Dallmann A, Liu XI, Burckart GJ, van den Anker J. Drug transporters expressed in the human placenta and models for studying maternal-Fetal drug transfer. Journal of Clinical Pharmacology. 2019;**59**(Suppl 1):S70-S81. DOI: 10.1002/jcph.1491

[8] Meah VL, Cockcroft JR, Backx K, et al. Cardiac output and related haemodynamics during pregnancy: A series of meta-analyses. Heart. 2016;**102**:518-526. DOI: 10.1136/heartjnl-2015-308476

[9] Costantine MM. Physiologic and pharmacokinetic changes in pregnancy. Frontiers in Pharmacology. 2014;**5**:65. DOI: 10.3389/fphar.2014.00065

[10] Hodge LS, Tracy TS. Alterations in drug disposition during pregnancy: Implications for drug therapy. Expert Opinion on Drug Metabolism & Toxicology. 2007;**3**:557-571. DOI: 10.1517/17425225.3.4.557

[11] Jeong H, Choi S, Song JW, et al. Regulation of UDP-glucuronosyltransferase (UGT) 1A1 by progesterone and its impact on labetalol elimination. Xenobiotica. 2008;**38**:62-75. DOI: 10.1080/00498250701744633

[12] Tan EK, Tan EL. Alterations in physiology and anatomy during pregnancy. Best Practice & Research. Clinical Obstetrics & Gynaecology. 2013;**27**:791-802. DOI: 10.1016/j.bpobgyn.2013.08.001

[13] Olmos-Ortiz A, Flores-Espinosa P, Díaz L, et al. Immunoendocrine dysregulation during gestational diabetes mellitus: The central role of the placenta. International Journal of Molecular Sciences. 2021;**22**:8087. DOI: 10.3390/ijms22158087

[14] Soma-Pillay P, Nelson-Piercy C, Tolppanen H, Mebazaa A. Physiological changes in pregnancy. Cardiovascular Journal of Africa. 2016;**27**:89-94. DOI: 10.5830/CVJA-2016-021

[15] Conrad KP, Davison JM. The renal circulation in normal pregnancy and preeclampsia: Is there a place for relaxin? American Journal of Physiology. Renal Physiology. 2014;**306**:F1121-F1135. DOI: 10.1152/ajprenal.00042.2014

[16] Cheung KL, Lafayette RA. Renal physiology of pregnancy. Advances in Chronic Kidney Disease. 2013;**20**:209-214. DOI: 10.1053/j.ackd.2013.01.012

[17] Feghali M, Venkataramanan R, Caritis S. Pharmacokinetics of drugs in pregnancy. Seminars in Perinatology. 2015;**39**:512-519. DOI: 10.1053/j.semperi.2015.08.003

[18] Bouazza N, Foissac F, Hirt D, et al. Methodological approaches to evaluate Fetal drug exposure. Current Pharmaceutical Design. 2019;**25**:496-504. DOI: 10.2174/1381612825666190319102812

[19] Bauchat J, Wong C. Chapter 36 - pain management during pregnancy and lactation. In: Essentials of Pain Medicine. Third ed. Saint Louis: W.B. Saunders; 2011. pp. 249-252

[20] Yates LM, Thomas SHL. Prescribing medicines in pregnancy. Medicine. 2016;**44**:438-443. DOI: 10.1016/j.mpmed.2016.04.012

[21] Buhimschi CS, Weiner CP. Medications in pregnancy and lactation: Part 1. Teratology. Obstetrics and Gynecology. 2009;**113**:166-188. DOI: 10.1097/AOG.0b013e31818d6788

[22] Alwan S, Chambers CD. Identifying Human Teratogens: An Update. Journal of Pediatric Genetics. 2015;**4**:39-41. DOI: 10.1055/s-0035-1556745

[23] Gupta RC. Reproductive and Developmental Toxicology. 2nd ed. San Diego, CA: Elsevier Academic Press; 2022

[24] Liu XI, Momper JD, Rakhmanina NY, et al. Physiologically based pharmacokinetic Modeling framework to predict neonatal pharmacokinetics of Transplacentally acquired Emtricitabine, Dolutegravir, and Raltegravir. Clinical Pharmacokinetics. 2021;**60**:795-809. DOI: 10.1007/s40262-020-00977-w

[25] Blanc WA, Johnson L. Studies on kernicterus; relationship with sulfonamide intoxication, report on kernicterus in rats with glucuronyl transferase deficiency and review of pathogenesis. Journal of Neuropathology and Experimental Neurology. 1959;**18**:165-187; discussion 187-189. DOI: 10.1097/00005072-195901000-00011

[26] Shintaku K, Hori S, Tsujimoto M, et al. Transplacental pharmacokinetics of diclofenac in perfused human placenta. Drug Metabolism and Disposition. 2009;**37**:962-968. DOI: 10.1124/dmd.108.024349

[27] Wiles JR, Isemann B, Ward LP, et al. Current management of neonatal abstinence syndrome secondary to intrauterine opioid exposure. The Journal of Pediatrics. 2014;**165**:440-446. DOI: 10.1016/j.jpeds.2014.05.010

[28] van den AJN. Neonatal abstinence syndrome: A never ending story! Journal of Pediatric and Neonatal Individualized Medicine (JPNIM). 2013;**2**:e020231-e020231. DOI: 10.7363/020231

[29] Levinson-Castiel R, Merlob P, Linder N, et al. Neonatal abstinence syndrome after in utero exposure to selective serotonin reuptake inhibitors in term infants. Archives of Pediatrics & Adolescent Medicine. 2006;**160**:173-176. DOI: 10.1001/archpedi.160.2.173

[30] Kellogg M, Meador KJ. Neurodevelopmental effects of antiepileptic drugs. Neurochemical Research. 2017;**42**:2065-2070. DOI: 10.1007/s11064-017-2262-4

[31] Lebin LG, Novick AM. Selective serotonin reuptake inhibitors (SSRIs) in pregnancy: An updated review on risks to mother, Fetus, and child. Current Psychiatry Reports. 2022;**24**:687-695. DOI: 10.1007/s11920-022-01372-x

[32] Shinohara H, Kodama H. Relationship between duration of crying/fussy behavior and actigraphic sleep measures in early infancy. Early Human Development. 2012;**88**:847-852. DOI: 10.1016/j.earlhumdev.2012.06.005

[33] Birru Talabi M, Miller R, Krishnamurti T. Medication decision making under uncertainty: Considering chronic disease and pregnancy potential. Seminars in Perinatology. 2025;**49**:152057. DOI: 10.1016/j.semperi.2025.152057

[34] Section on Breastfeeding. Breastfeeding and the use of human milk. Pediatrics. 2012;**129**:e827-e841. DOI: 10.1542/peds.2011-3552

[35] Gomez-Casado G, Alonso-Titos J, Gonzalez-Mesa E, Ortega-Gomez A. Compatibility of post-kidney transplant immunosuppression therapy with lactation. Journal of Clinical Medicine. 2025;**14**:2364. DOI: 10.3390/jcm14072364

[36] Spencer JP, Thomas S, Trondsen Pawlowski RH. Medication safety in breastfeeding. American Family Physician. 2022;**106**:638-644

[37] Morze K, Szałek E, Waszyk-Nowaczyk M. Minding the gap. Drug-related problems among breastfeeding women. Frontiers in Pharmacology. 2025;**16**:1542269. DOI: 10.3389/fphar.2025.1542269

[38] What Barriers and Facilitators to.... HRB Open Research. Available from: https://hrbopenresearch.org/articles/8-53 [Accessed: August 1, 2025]

[39] Pan X, Rowland Yeo K. Addressing drug safety of maternal therapy during breastfeeding using physiologically-based pharmacokinetic modeling. CPT: Pharmacometrics & Systems Pharmacology. 2022;**11**:535-539. DOI: 10.1002/psp4.12802

[40] Prednisone. In: Drugs and Lactation Database (LactMed®). Bethesda (MD): National Institute of Child Health and Human Development; 2006. Available from: https://www.ncbi.nlm.nih.gov/books/NBK501077/

[41] Sodium Iodide I 131. In: Drugs and Lactation Database (LactMed®). Bethesda (MD): National Institute of Child Health and Human Development; 2006. Available from: https://www.ncbi.nlm.nih.gov/books/NBK501563/

[42] Gallium Citrate Ga 67. In: Drugs and Lactation Database (LactMed®). Bethesda (MD): National Institute of Child Health and Human Development; 2006. Available from: https://www.ncbi.nlm.nih.gov/books/NBK501557/

[43] Theurey P, Vial G, Fontaine E, et al. Reduced lactic acidosis risk with Imeglimin: Comparison with metformin. Physiological Reports. 2022;**10**:e15151. DOI: 10.14814/phy2.15151

[44] Labetalol. In: Drugs and Lactation Database (LactMed®). Bethesda (MD): National Institute of Child Health and Human Development; 2006. Available from: https://www.ncbi.nlm.nih.gov/books/NBK501151/

[45] Sertraline. In: Drugs and Lactation Database (LactMed®). Bethesda (MD): National Institute of Child Health and Human Development; 2006. Available from: https://www.ncbi.nlm.nih.gov/books/NBK501191/

[46] Paulzen M. Psychotropic Medication and Breastfeeding – Yes – No – Maybe?

[47] Oladapo OT, Fawole B. Treatments for suppression of lactation. Cochrane Database of Systematic Reviews. 2012;**2012**:CD005937. DOI: 10.1002/14651858.CD005937.pub3

[48] Stopping your Milk Supply (Lactation Suppression). Australian Breastfeeding Association. Available from: https://www.breastfeeding.asn.au/resources/stopping-milk-supply [Accessed: August 1, 2025]

[49] Blattner CM, Danesh M, Safaee M, Murase JE. Understanding the new FDA pregnancy and lactation labeling rules. International Journal of Women's Dermatology. 2016;**2**:5-7. DOI: 10.1016/j.ijwd.2015.12.005

[50] Brucker MC, King TL. The 2015 US Food and Drug Administration pregnancy and lactation Labeling rule. Journal of Midwifery & Women's Health. 2017;**62**:308-316. DOI: 10.1111/jmwh.12611

[51] Nordeng H. Drug utilization in pregnant women. In: Drug Utilization Research: Methods and Applications. Chichester, UK: John Wiley & Sons, Ltd; 2016. pp. 240-247

[52] Donald S, Sharples K, Barson D, et al. Patterns of prescription medicine dispensing before and during pregnancy in New Zealand, 2005-2015. PLoS One. 2020;**15**:e0234153. DOI: 10.1371/journal.pone.0234153

[53] Donald S, Sharples K, Barson D, et al. Prescription medicines with potential for foetal harm: Dispensing before and during pregnancy in New Zealand, 2005-2015. European Journal of Clinical Pharmacology. 2020;**76**:887-896. DOI: 10.1007/s00228-020-02868-2

[54] Houben E, Te Winkel B, Steegers EAP, Herings RMC. Dutch trends in the use of potentially harmful medication during pregnancy. British Journal of Clinical Pharmacology. 2020;**86**:2377-2392. DOI: 10.1111/bcp.14341

[55] Larcin L, Lona M, Karakaya G, et al. Using administrative healthcare database records to study trends in prescribed medication dispensed during pregnancy in Belgium from 2003 to 2017. Pharmacoepidemiology and Drug Safety. 2021;**30**:1224-1232. DOI: 10.1002/pds.5299

[56] Havard A, Barbieri S, Hanly M, et al. Medications used disproportionately during pregnancy: Priorities for research on the risks and benefits of medications when used during pregnancy. Pharmacoepidemiology and Drug Safety. 2021;**30**:53-64. DOI: 10.1002/pds.5131

[57] Lupattelli A, Spigset O, Twigg MJ, et al. Medication use in pregnancy: A cross-sectional, multinational web-based study. BMJ Open. 2014;**4**:e004365. DOI: 10.1136/bmjopen-2013-004365

[58] Lupattelli A, Picinardi M, Cantarutti A, Nordeng H. Use and intentional avoidance of prescribed medications in pregnancy: A cross-sectional, web-based study among 926 women in Italy. International Journal of Environmental Research and Public Health. 2020;**17**:3830. DOI: 10.3390/ijerph17113830

[59] NHS Maternal Use of SSRIs Neonatal Clinical Guideline V4.1. 2024

[60] Corti S, Pileri P, Mazzocco MI, et al. Neonatal outcomes in maternal depression in relation to intrauterine drug exposure. Frontiers in Pediatrics. 2019;7:309. DOI: 10.3389/fped.2019.00309

[61] Gao S-Y, Wu Q-J, Sun C, et al. Selective serotonin reuptake inhibitor use during early pregnancy and congenital malformations: A systematic review and meta-analysis of cohort studies of more than 9 million births. BMC Medicine. 2018;**16**:205. DOI: 10.1186/s12916-018-1193-5

[62] Zhang T-N, Gao S-Y, Shen Z-Q, et al. Use of selective serotonin-reuptake inhibitors in the first trimester and risk of cardiovascular-related malformations: A meta-analysis of cohort studies. Scientific Reports. 2017;7:43085. DOI: 10.1038/srep43085

[63] Güngör BB, Öztürk N, Atar AÖ, Aydın N. Comparison of the groups treated with mirtazapine and selective serotonine reuptake inhibitors with respect to birth outcomes and severity of psychiatric disorder. Psychiatry and Clinical Psychopharmacology. 2019;**29**:822-831. DOI: 10.1080/24750573.2019.1673936

[64] Hwang YM, Roper RT, Piekos SN, et al. Timing of selective serotonin reuptake inhibitor use and risk for preterm birth and related adverse events: With a consideration of the COVID-19 pandemic period. The Journal of Maternal-Fetal & Neonatal Medicine. 2024;**37**:2313364. DOI: 10.1080/14767058.2024.2313364

[65] Domingues RR, Fricke HP, Sheftel CM, et al. Effect of low and high doses of two selective serotonin reuptake inhibitors on pregnancy outcomes and neonatal mortality. Toxics. 2022;**10**:11. DOI: 10.3390/toxics10010011

[66] Andrade C. Epilepsy, antiepileptic drugs, and adverse pregnancy outcomes, 2: Major congenital malformations with antiepileptic drug monotherapy. The Journal of Clinical Psychiatry. 2024;**85**:24f15432. DOI: 10.4088/JCP.24f15432

[67] Hope OA, Harris KM. Management of epilepsy during pregnancy and lactation. BMJ. 2023;**382**:e074630. DOI: 10.1136/bmj-2022-074630

[68] Hernández-Díaz S, Smith CR, Shen A, et al. Comparative safety of antiepileptic drugs during pregnancy. Neurology. 2012;**78**:1692-1699. DOI: 10.1212/WNL.0b013e3182574f39

[69] Tomson T, Battino D, Perucca E. Teratogenicity of antiepileptic drugs. Current Opinion in Neurology. 2019;**32**:246-252. DOI: 10.1097/WCO.0000000000000659

[70] (pdf) Pharmacological Safety of Antiepileptic Drugs in Pregnant and Lactating Women. ResearchGate

[71] Nucera B, Brigo F, Trinka E, Kalss G. Treatment and care of women with epilepsy before, during, and after pregnancy: A practical guide. Therapeutic Advances in Neurological Disorders. 2022;**15**:17562864221101687. DOI: 10.1177/17562864221101687

[72] Pennell PB, Gidal BE, Sabers A, et al. Pharmacology of antiepileptic drugs during pregnancy and lactation. Epilepsy & Behavior. 2007;**11**:263-269. DOI: 10.1016/j.yebeh.2007.08.018

[73] Veroniki AA, Rios P, Cogo E, et al. Comparative safety of antiepileptic

drugs for neurological development in children exposed during pregnancy and breast feeding: A systematic review and network meta-analysis. BMJ Open. 2017;**7**:e017248. DOI: 10.1136/bmjopen-2017-017248

[74] Pennell PB. Use of antiepileptic drugs during pregnancy: Evolving concepts. Neurotherapeutics. 2016;**13**:811-820. DOI: 10.1007/s13311-016-0464-0

[75] Karanam A, Pennell PB, French JA, et al. Lamotrigine clearance increases by 5 weeks gestational age: Relationship to estradiol concentrations and gestational age. Annals of Neurology. 2018;**84**:556-563. DOI: 10.1002/ana.25321

[76] Arfman IJ, Wammes-van der Heijden EA, Ter Horst PGJ, et al. Therapeutic drug monitoring of antiepileptic drugs in women with epilepsy before, during, and after pregnancy. Clinical Pharmacokinetics. 2020;**59**:427-445. DOI: 10.1007/s40262-019-00845-2

[77] Bookstaver PB, Bland CM, Griffin B, et al. A review of antibiotic use in pregnancy. Pharmacotherapy. 2015;**35**:1052 1062. DOI: 10.1002/phar.1649

[78] Nguyen J, Madonia V, Bland CM, et al. A review of antibiotic safety in pregnancy-2025 update. Pharmacotherapy. 2025;**45**:227-237. DOI: 10.1002/phar.70010

[79] Nahum GG, Uhl K, Kennedy DL. Antibiotic use in pregnancy and lactation: What is and is not known about teratogenic and toxic risks. Obstetrics and Gynecology. 2006;**107**:1120-1138. DOI: 10.1097/01.AOG.0000216197.26783.b5

[80] Yu PA, Tran EL, Parker CM, et al. Safety of antimicrobials during pregnancy: A systematic review of antimicrobials considered for treatment and Postexposure prophylaxis of plague. Clinical Infectious Diseases. 2020;**70**:S37-S50. DOI: 10.1093/cid/ciz1231

[81] Alemu BK, Wang CC, Li L, et al. Effect of preconception antibiotics exposure on female reproductive health and pregnancy outcomes: A systematic review and meta-analysis. EClinicalMedicine. 2024;**78**:102935. DOI: 10.1016/j.eclinm.2024.102935

[82] Kuperman AA, Koren O. Antibiotic use during pregnancy: How bad is it? BMC Medicine. 2016;**14**:91. DOI: 10.1186/s12916-016-0636-0

[83] Ledger WJ, Blaser MJ. Are we using too many antibiotics during pregnancy? BJOG. 2013;**120**:1450-1452. DOI: 10.1111/1471-0528.12371

[84] Cantarutti A, Rea F, Franchi M, et al. Use of antibiotic treatment in pregnancy and the risk of several neonatal outcomes: A population-based study. International Journal of Environmental Research and Public Health. 2021;**18**:12621. DOI: 10.3390/ijerph182312621

[85] Zhang M, Differding MK, Benjamin-Neelon SE, et al. Association of prenatal antibiotics with measures of infant adiposity and the gut microbiome. Annals of Clinical Microbiology and Antimicrobials. 2019;**18**:18. DOI: 10.1186/s12941-019-0318-9

[86] Brocklehurst P, Gordon A, Heatley E, Milan SJ. Antibiotics for treating bacterial vaginosis in pregnancy. Cochrane Database of Systematic Reviews. 31 Jan 2013;**2013**(1):CD000262. DOI: 10.1002/14651858.CD000262.pub4

[87] Ehsan F. Hussein, & Haider Qassim Raheem. Antibiotic susceptibility

patterns of Staphylococcus aureus isolated from pregnant women with urinary tract infections. Journal of Population Therapeutics and Clinical Pharmacology. 2023;**30**(1):218-224

[88] Ray-Griffith SL, Wendel MP, Stowe ZN, Magann EF. Chronic pain during pregnancy: A review of the literature. International Journal of Women's Health. 2018;**10**:153-164. DOI: 10.2147/IJWH.S151845

[89] Zafeiri A, Mitchell RT, Hay DC, Fowler PA. Over-the-counter analgesics during pregnancy: A comprehensive review of global prevalence and offspring safety. Human Reproduction Update. 2021;**27**:67-95. DOI: 10.1093/humupd/dmaa042

[90] Ghorpade SS, Shetty PN, Bonanthaya K, Rao D. Isolated Paramedian cleft of lower LIP: A rare entity. The Cleft Palate-Craniofacial Journal. 2024;**61**:1919-1924. DOI: 10.1177/10556656231185971

[91] Antonucci R, Zaffanello M, Puxeddu E, et al. Use of non-steroidal anti-inflammatory drugs in pregnancy: Impact on the fetus and newborn. Current Drug Metabolism. 2012;**13**:474-490. DOI: 10.2174/138920012800166607

[92] Carvajal AB, Ayala N, Duran N, Cubides Munevar AM, Guerrero N. Effects of nonsteroid antiinflammatory drugs on pregnant women and the fetus: A systematic review of literature [Preprint]. 2023. Preprints.org

[93] Shahid S. Beyond pain relief: The unseen consequences of NSAIDs misuse in pregnancy. The Journal of the Pakistan Medical Association. 2025;**75**:177. DOI: 10.47391/JPMA.20740

[94] Bloor M, Paech M. Nonsteroidal anti-inflammatory drugs during pregnancy and the initiation of lactation. Anesthesia and Analgesia. 2013;**116**:1063-1075. DOI: 10.1213/ANE.0b013e31828a4b54

[95] Källén B, Reis M. Ongoing pharmacological Management of Chronic Pain in pregnancy. Drugs. 2016;**76**:915-924. DOI: 10.1007/s40265-016-0582-3

[96] Nunge RA, Kendle AM, Alwan S. Pain medication use during pregnancy. Seminars in Perinatology. 2025;**49**:152074. DOI: 10.1016/j.semperi.2025.152074

[97] Crescioli G, Lombardi N, Vannacci A. Editorial: Safety of drugs and CAM products in pregnancy and breastfeeding: Evidence from clinical toxicology. Frontiers in Pharmacology. 2023;**14**:1340283. DOI: 10.3389/fphar.2023.1340283

[98] Ahmed M, Hwang JH, Choi S, Han D. Safety classification of herbal medicines used among pregnant women in Asian countries: A systematic review. BMC Complementary and Alternative Medicine. 2017;**17**:489. DOI: 10.1186/s12906-017-1995-6

[99] Bernstein N, Akram M, Yaniv-Bachrach Z, Daniyal M. Is it safe to consume traditional medicinal plants during pregnancy? Phytotherapy Research. 2021;**35**:1908-1924. DOI: 10.1002/ptr.6935

[100] Balarastaghi S, Delirrad M, Jafari A, et al. Potential benefits versus hazards of herbal therapy during pregnancy; a systematic review of available literature. Phytotherapy Research. 2022;**36**:824-841. DOI: 10.1002/ptr.7363

[101] Sarecka-Hujar B, Szulc-Musioł B. Herbal medicines-are they effective and safe during pregnancy? Pharmaceutics. 2022;**14**:171. DOI: 10.3390/pharmaceutics14010171

[102] Heitmann K, Havnen GC, Holst L, Nordeng H. Pregnancy outcomes after prenatal exposure to echinacea: The Norwegian mother and child cohort study. European Journal of Clinical Pharmacology. 2016;**72**:623-630. DOI: 10.1007/s00228-016-2021-5

[103] NCCIH. Evening primrose oil: Usefulness and safety. In: NCCIH. Available from: https://www.nccih.nih.gov/health/evening-primrose-oil

[104] Xiong Y, Liu C, Li M, et al. The use of Chinese herbal medicines throughout the pregnancy life course and their safety profiles: A population-based cohort study. American Journal of Obstetrics & Gynecology MFM. 2023;**5**:100907. DOI: 10.1016/j.ajogmf.2023.100907

[105] Bettiol A, Lombardi N, Marconi E, et al. The use of complementary and alternative medicines during breastfeeding: Results from the herbal supplements in breastfeeding InvesTigation (HaBIT) study. British Journal of Clinical Pharmacology. 2018;**84**:2040-2047. DOI: 10.1111/bcp.13639

[106] Bettiol A, Lombardi N, Marconi E, et al. The impact of previous pregnancy loss on lactating Behaviors and use of herbal medicines during breastfeeding: A post hoc analysis of the herbal supplements in breastfeeding InvesTigation (HaBIT). Evidence-Based Complementary and Alternative Medicine. 2018;**2018**:1035875. DOI: 10.1155/2018/1035875

[107] Gallo E, Lucenteforte E, Firenzuoli F, et al. Herbalists' perception of risks involving commonly sold medicinal plants in Italy. Complementary Therapies in Medicine. 2014;**22**:81-86. DOI: 10.1016/j.ctim.2013.12.002

[108] Mannucci C, Dante G, Miroddi M, et al. Vigilance on use of drugs, herbal products, and food supplements during pregnancy: Focus on fosfomycin. The Journal of Maternal-Fetal & Neonatal Medicine. 2019;**32**:125-128. DOI: 10.1080/14767058.2017.1373761

[109] Lynch MM, Amoozegar JB, McClure EM, et al. Improving safe use of medications during pregnancy: The roles of patients, physicians, and pharmacists. Qualitative Health Research. 2017;**27**:2071-2080. DOI: 10.1177/1049732317732027

[110] Goruntla N, Pandey P, Gullakunta A, et al. Knowledge, attitude and practice of community pharmacists on medication safety during pregnancy: A cross-sectional study. International Journal of Pharmaceutical Investigation. 2025;**9**(4):215-219

[111] Kelty E, Hansen M, Randall S, et al. Use of privacy-preserving record linkage to examine the dispensing of pharmaceutical benefits scheme medicines to pregnant women in Western Australia. Pharmacoepidemiology and Drug Safety. 2024;**33**:e5845. DOI: 10.1002/pds.5845

[112] Spehar SM, Albert-Stone E, Davis MB. Cardiac medications in obstetric patients. Current Opinion in Cardiology. 2023;**38**:266-274. DOI: 10.1097/HCO.0000000000001039

[113] Subramanian A, Azcoaga-Lorenzo A, Anand A, et al. Polypharmacy during pregnancy and associated risk factors: A retrospective analysis of 577 medication exposures among 1.5 million pregnancies in the UK, 2000-2019. BMC Medicine. 2023;**21**:21. DOI: 10.1186/s12916-022-02722-5

[114] Noda A, Obara T, Shirota M, et al. Medication use before and during pregnancy in Japan: The Tohoku medical megabank project birth and

three-generation cohort study. European Journal of Clinical Pharmacology. 2024;**80**:1171-1180. DOI: 10.1007/s00228-024-03685-7

[115] Kim J-W, Suh C-H. The safety of medications during pregnancy and lactation in patients with inflammatory rheumatic diseases. European Medical Journal. 2021. DOI: 10.33590/emj/21-00017

[116] Sinclair SM, Miller RK, Chambers C, Cooper EM. Medication safety during pregnancy: Improving evidence-based practice. Journal of Midwifery & Women's Health. 2016;**61**:52-67. DOI: 10.1111/jmwh.12358

[117] Alexe A, Garg A, Kovacs B, et al. Regulations governing medicines for maternal and neonatal health: A landscape assessment. Therapeutic Innovation & Regulatory Science. 2024;**58**:242-257. DOI: 10.1007/s43441-023-00593-3

[118] Ahmed SM, Sundby J, Aragaw YA, Abebe F. Self-medication and safety profile of medicines used among pregnant women in a tertiary teaching Hospital in Jimma, Ethiopia: A cross-sectional study. International Journal of Environmental Research and Public Health. 2020;**17**:3993. DOI: 10.3390/ijerph17113993

[119] Ghalandari N, Dolhain RJEM, Hazes JMW, et al. Intrauterine exposure to biologics in inflammatory autoimmune diseases: A systematic review. Drugs. 2020;**80**:1699-1722. DOI: 10.1007/s40265-020-01376-y

[120] Wood ME, Andrade SE, Toh S. Safe expectations: Current state and future directions for medication safety in pregnancy research. Clinical Therapeutics. 2019;**41**:2467-2476. DOI: 10.1016/j.clinthera.2019.08.016

[121] Wood ME, Lapane KL, van Gelder MMHJ, et al. Making fair comparisons in pregnancy medication safety studies: An overview of advanced methods for confounding control. Pharmacoepidemiology and Drug Safety. 2018;**27**:140-147. DOI: 10.1002/pds.4336

[122] Clowse MEB, Feldman SR, Isaacs JD, et al. Pregnancy outcomes in the Tofacitinib safety databases for rheumatoid arthritis and psoriasis. Drug Safety. 2016;**39**:755-762. DOI: 10.1007/s40264-016-0431-z

[123] Hollestelle MJ, van der Graaf R, Hartman SD, et al. A learning healthcare system for pregnant and breastfeeding women: What do women during preconception, pregnancy, and nursing think? - a qualitative study : A contribution from the ConcePTION project. BMC Pregnancy and Childbirth. 2022;**22**:334. DOI: 10.1186/s12884-022-04675-2

[124] Byrne JJ, Saucedo AM, Spong CY. Evaluation of drug labels following the 2015 pregnancy and lactation Labeling rule. JAMA Network Open. 2020;**3**:e2015094. DOI: 10.1001/jamanetworkopen.2020.15094

[125] Keller MS, Mosadeghi S, Cohen ER, et al. Reproductive health and medication concerns for patients with inflammatory bowel disease: Thematic and quantitative analysis using social listening. Journal of Medical Internet Research. 2018;**20**:e206. DOI: 10.2196/jmir.9870

[126] Casey E, Velez MP, Gaudet L, Brogly SB. The use, perceptions and knowledge of safety of over-the-counter medications during pregnancy in a Canadian population. Womens Health (Lond). 2023;**19**:17455057231199394. DOI: 10.1177/17455057231199394

[127] Zitoun N, Campbell MK, Matsui D, Garcia-Bournissen F. Prospective

evaluation of pregnancy outcomes after gestational exposure to prazosin. British Journal of Clinical Pharmacology. Nov 2023;**89**(11):3324-3329. DOI: 10.1111/bcp.15829

[128] Pedersen LH, Petersen OB, Nørgaard M, et al. Linkage between the Danish National Health Service Prescription Database, the Danish Fetal medicine database, and other Danish registries as a tool for the study of drug safety in pregnancy. Clinical Epidemiology. 2016;**8**:91-95. DOI: 10.2147/CLEP.S98139

[129] Pijpers EL, Kreijkamp-Kaspers S, McGuire TM, et al. Women's questions about medicines in pregnancy - an analysis of calls to an Australian national medicines call Centre. The Australian & New Zealand Journal of Obstetrics & Gynaecology. 2017;**57**:334-341. DOI: 10.1111/ajo.12531

[130] Palmsten K, Hernández-Díaz S, Chambers CD, et al. The Most commonly dispensed prescription medications among pregnant women enrolled in the U.S. Medicaid program. Obstetrics and Gynecology. 2015;**126**:465-473. DOI: 10.1097/AOG.0000000000000982

[131] de Waard M, Blomjous BS, Hol MLF, et al. Medication use during pregnancy and lactation in a Dutch population. Journal of Human Lactation. 2019;**35**:154-164. DOI: 10.1177/0890334418775630

Chapter 4

Inappropriate Medication Use in Geriatric Patients: Factors and Management

Ahmet Çakır and Hasan Memiş

Abstract

In older adults, age-related physiological, anatomical, and metabolic changes, compounded by issues of multimorbidity and polypharmacy, substantially heighten the risk of potentially inappropriate medication (PIM) utilization. PIM, characterized by drug use in which risks surpass benefits, represents a key factor contributing to adverse drug events (ADEs), potential drug-drug interactions (pDDIs), hospitalizations, frailty, and increased healthcare expenditures. PIM arises from multiple factors, including patient-related issues, such as polypharmacy, multimorbidity, cognitive decline, poor adherence, and self-medication; physician-related contributors, such as prescribing cascades, insufficient medication review, and fragmented care; and system-level barriers, such as inadequate medication management programs, limited consultation time, communication gaps, and financial constraints. Among the major consequences of PIM are ADEs, increased risk of falls, higher hospitalization rates, and escalating healthcare expenditures. Several management strategies have been proposed to minimize these risks. Key clinical interventions involve structured medication review and reconciliation, deprescribing, individualized prescribing guided by clinical decision support tools, and measures to enhance adherence. Interventions at the system level, such as comprehensive medication management programs, pharmacist-conducted reviews, collaborative interprofessional approaches, and the incorporation of computerized decision support tools, are vital for promoting safe prescribing. In parallel, patient and caregiver participation, reinforced by education and reporting of adverse events, significantly contributes to the reduction of PIMs. Effectively minimizing PIMs demands a holistic and interdisciplinary framework. Enhancing interprofessional collaboration, supporting patient-centered care initiatives, and examining the long-term outcomes of such strategies are critical for improving pharmacotherapy and healthcare quality in the geriatric population.

Keywords: adverse drug events, deprescribing, geriatric patients, polypharmacy, potentially inappropriate medication

1. Introduction

The aging process not only predisposes individuals to chronic diseases but also brings about anatomical, physiological, and metabolic changes that require careful consideration in medical treatment and pharmacological interventions [1]. These changes have significant implications, as older adults frequently face chronic illnesses, frailty, and cognitive decline, placing substantial demands on healthcare systems and resources [2]. The global increase in the elderly population has made the issues of multimorbidity and polypharmacy more prominent. Inappropriate medication use (IMU) is defined as the use of medicines whose risks outweigh their benefits when safer alternatives are available [3]. In a recent study, the prevalence of potentially inappropriate medication (PIM) use in outpatient services worldwide was estimated to be 36.7% [4]. Polypharmacy in the elderly increases the risk of inappropriate drug use, which brings with it certain challenges for the healthcare system [5]. In this context, IMU, adverse drug events (ADEs), and controlling medication costs have become key challenges in healthcare delivery [6]. Specifically, the burden of polypharmacy has been linked to increased healthcare costs, higher risk of potential drug-drug interactions (pDDIs), poor medication adherence, diminished functional capacity, and the development of multiple geriatric syndromes [7]. There are many factors associated with the presence of IMU in older adults. These include mainly patient-related factors, physician-related factors, and system-related factors [8]. All these factors should be thoroughly investigated and addressed through appropriate interventions to minimize the occurrence of IMU. A variety of well-validated tools and criteria have been developed to facilitate the detection and management of IMUs in the elderly population. Among the most commonly employed tools are the american geriatrics society (AGS) Beers Criteria [9], TIME Criteria [10], PRISCUS List [11], START (Screening Tool to Alert to Right Treatment)-STOPP (Screening Tool of Older Persons' Prescriptions) Criteria [12], FORTA (Fit fOR The Aged) List [13], Chinese PIM criteria [14], and the European Union (EU) (7)-PIM List [15], all of which aim to guide appropriate prescribing practices in older adults. Many of these criteria have been developed on a country-by-country basis and have national characteristics. Using these criteria, undesirable effects that may occur in the presence of PIM can be eliminated.

2. Factors causing inappropriate medication use

The combination of age-related physiological alterations, multiple clinical conditions, and social complexities renders older adults highly susceptible to adverse health outcomes. Therefore, factors affecting the presence of IMU in this population negatively affect the quality of life. The main contributors include:

2.1 Patient-related factors

Patient-related factors causing IMU include polypharmacy, multiple chronic conditions, physiological changes with aging, cognitive decline and sensory impairment, self-medication, and poor adherence.

2.1.1 Polypharmacy

While there is no universally accepted definition, polypharmacy is commonly described as the regular use of five or more medications by an individual, encompassing prescription drugs, over-the-counter products, as well as traditional and complementary therapies [16]. In addition, the term hyperpolypharmacy is defined as the simultaneous intake of 10 or more medications [17]. Polypharmacy often stems from the need to manage multiple comorbidities, the involvement of various healthcare providers, a lack of coordinated care, and the increased accessibility of over-the-counter medications. This phenomenon is further exacerbated by the rising degree of medical specialization within healthcare systems, frequently resulting in complex therapeutic regimens implemented without interdisciplinary consensus. Although concurrent pharmacological treatment may be clinically justified in individuals with multiple conditions, the cumulative drug burden can lead to organ dysfunction, drug-drug and drug-disease interactions, medication nonadherence, increased morbidity and mortality, diminished quality of life, and elevated healthcare expenditures due to IMU [18]. Polypharmacy is associated with an elevated risk of ADEs, harmful pDDIs, and reduced medication adherence, as well as increased rates of hospitalization, falls, frailty, cognitive decline, and mortality among geriatric patients [19]. In developed countries, an estimated 30–40% of individuals over the age of 65 use five or more medications, while approximately 12% take 10 or more different drugs [20]. While polypharmacy is linked to adverse outcomes in older adults, aging itself influences the relationship between medication use and clinical effects. Age-related alterations in pharmacokinetics and body composition impact drug metabolism, clearance, and distribution, increasing susceptibility to adverse drug reactions (ADRs) [21]. Age, polypharmacy, and the presence of specific chronic conditions were identified as independent determinants associated with PIMs and pDDIs [22]. Addressing these factors through individualized medication management strategies, renal function-based dose optimization, and the avoidance of unnecessary polypharmacy may contribute to risk mitigation. In the geriatric population, the use of PIMs is associated with a heightened risk of unplanned hospitalizations, particularly in individuals receiving polypharmacy, underscoring the need for caution when prescribing PIMs to older adults [23]. Encouraging the rational use of medications through multidisciplinary collaboration, conducting regular pharmacotherapy reviews, and personalizing treatment to meet individual patient needs may reduce mortality and mitigate the risks linked to polypharmacy [24]. Pharmacist-led deprescribing interventions in older adults can substantially reduce the use of PIMs, thereby mitigating polypharmacy, with potentially greater effectiveness when implemented within a multidisciplinary care framework.

2.1.2 Multiple chronic conditions

In the geriatric population, susceptibility to diseases increases with changing physiology with age, and multimorbidity may be observed in these patients compared to younger adults. The term multimorbidity refers to the presence of at least two chronic diseases within the same patient [25]. Among older individuals, the combination of multiple diseases may interact in a super-additive manner, exacerbating declines in functional status, compromising quality of life, and shortening life expectancy, which collectively contribute to complex health and care requirements [26, 27]. Advanced age is the most significant determinant of multimorbidity, with prevalence rates reaching approximately 90% in those aged 85 years and above [28]. Hypertension is the most common disease among the elderly, followed by osteoarthritis and diabetes mellitus. More than one drug may be required to treat such diseases, so some undesirable drug-related problems such as pDDIs and ADEs may occur during treatment [29]. However, in the presence of underlying diseases (e.g., renal and hepatic insufficiency), the metabolism of drugs used for treatment changes significantly. Another challenge in the management of chronic conditions is the difficulty of medication administration in patients with impairments, such as visual or cognitive decline and dysphagia [30]. The aging process is universal yet heterogeneous. Recognizing physiological changes associated with aging, including diminished vision and hearing, delayed reaction times, and impaired balance, enables patients and caregivers to better manage risks, make appropriate healthcare decisions, and reduce the likelihood of falls and medication-related complications. In cases of multimorbidity, a comprehensive geriatric assessment should serve as the first step, enabling the systematic identification of all existing health conditions and the implementation of tailored interventions. Subsequently, continuous and periodic evaluation of disease status and therapeutic regimens is necessary, as it plays a pivotal role in recognizing and preventing IMU [31]. A multidisciplinary approach may be required in this process.

2.1.3 Physiological changes

Physiological changes with age can significantly alter the course of the disease in the elderly. In older adults, physiological changes occur in virtually all solid organ systems as a natural consequence of aging, leading collectively to a decline in physiological reserve and reduced capacity to cope with stressors [32]. The changes that drugs undergo in the body may differ due to some pharmacokinetic and pharmacodynamic changes. For instance, age-related alterations in body composition reduce the volume of distribution of water-soluble drugs, resulting in higher serum concentrations in older adults. In elderly individuals, decreased renal function, particularly decreased glomerular filtration rate, affects the clearance of many water-soluble drugs. Such reductions in renal excretion may result in toxic drug levels [33]. The aging process involves structural and functional alterations across all organ systems, resulting in a reduced homeostatic capacity. Consequently, individualized treatment that accounts for the impact of these changes on pharmacotherapy in older adults is essential.

2.1.4 Cognitive impairment

Compared with younger populations, older adults appear to have an increased susceptibility to the development of cognitive impairment due to pharmacological exposure, a phenomenon attributable to age-related physiological changes, altered pharmacokinetics and pharmacodynamics, and a higher prevalence of polypharmacy [34]. Cognitive dysfunction denotes impairments across multiple domains, including attentional capacity, visual and auditory information processing, executive problem-solving abilities, processing speed, and motor performance [35]. Approximately one-quarter of older individuals are affected by cognitive impairment or dementia, with prevalence rising to almost 40% in those aged 80 and over [36]. The presence of PIM in the elderly is a factor that should not be ignored and may increase the severity of cognitive disorders. Drug-induced cognitive impairment refers to a decline in cognitive functioning attributable primarily to pharmacological agents. This adverse effect on cognitive abilities may result from the use of both central nervous system (CNS)-active and non-CNS-active medications [37]. The pharmacological classes most frequently implicated in drug-induced cognitive impairment encompass anticholinergic agents, hypnotics and sedatives, antipsychotics, opioid analgesics, antiparkinsonian medications, antidepressants, antiepileptic drugs, nonsteroidal anti-inflammatory drugs (NSAIDs), and proton pump inhibitors (PPIs) [34, 37]. Patients with cognitive impairment often have difficulty following medication administration's instructions or may experience treatment disruptions because they cannot remember to take the medication. Managing patients with cognitive impairment necessitates a critical evaluation of pharmacological agents that may contribute to its onset or progression. Establishing a causal link with a single drug is often difficult; thus, medications with a high risk of cognitive adverse effects should be closely monitored.

2.1.5 Self-medication

Another patient-related factor causing IMU is the use of over-the-counter or herbal medications, which is referred to as patient self-medication. It states that self-medication means selecting and using medications for self-diagnosed ailments or diseases [38]. This can become a bigger problem when doctors are not aware of it because these medications can cause changes in the effects of the medications the patient uses regularly. Individuals often use medications based solely on their own knowledge and experience rather than seeking medical advice or a prescription. This practice is particularly concerning in the care of older adults, where it may also involve the use of medications prescribed for family members [39]. This practice entails multiple risks for individuals, including misdiagnosis, delayed medical consultation, inappropriate treatment, unrecognized pharmacological hazards, adverse drug reactions, drug-drug and drug-food interactions, dosing errors, and risks of misuse or dependence. At the community level, inappropriate self-medication contributes to drug-related morbidity and unnecessary healthcare expenditures.

2.1.6 Poor adherence

The effectiveness of a medication depends on its use in accordance with the physician's instructions, highlighting the critical role of treatment adherence. Adherence to treatment is defined as the degree to which an individual's behaviors—such as medication intake, dietary practices, and lifestyle modifications—correspond with the recommendations agreed upon with a healthcare provider [40]. Nonadherence rates to drug treatment in elderly patients with comorbidities have been reported as 31–53% [41, 42]. In elderly patients, treatment adherence is affected by various factors, such as side effects, memory impairment, challenges in medication management, socioeconomic conditions, health status, and inadequate communication with healthcare providers [43, 44]. The validated Morisky Medication Adherence Scale, which measures adherence on a 3-level ordinal scale, can be used to assess adherence [45]. Poor adherence to prescribed medications among older adults is a significant public health concern. Therefore, evaluating the factors that influence nonadherence is essential for improving health outcomes, minimizing medication waste, and reducing healthcare costs. Potentially inappropriate medications represent an important determinant of medication adherence in this population.

2.2 Physician-related factors

Physician-related factors contributing to IMU include prescribing cascades, inadequate medication review, prescribing habits, and fragmented care.

2.2.1 Prescribing cascade

Another simple but often overlooked cause of IMU is prescribing cascades. A prescribing cascade occurs when the side effects of a medication prompt the prescription of an additional drug to counteract or prevent those effects [46]. An unintended prescribing cascade arises when an adverse drug reaction is mistaken for a new medical condition, leading to the prescription of additional medications to address the resulting symptoms. For instance, pretibial edema caused by calcium channel blockers (CCBs) may be misinterpreted as a sign of congestive heart failure, resulting in the inappropriate prescription of a loop diuretic rather than switching to an alternative antihypertensive, such as lercanidipine, to alleviate the edema [47, 48]. In this example, prescribing another drug to treat another side effect that would be caused by the loop diuretic prescribed could extend this chain of incorrect prescribing. To prevent this situation, it may be necessary to take a complete medication history from patients and consider any medication-related side effects.

2.2.2 Inadequate medication review

One of the most effective strategies for minimizing therapeutic complexity and reducing the use of PIMs is the systematic review of prescribed drugs. Medication review is defined as a structured evaluation of a patient's medications with the aim of optimizing drug use and improving health outcomes, which includes the identification of drug-related problems and the recommendation of appropriate interventions [49]. It is essential to review patients' existing medication records not only prior to initiating new prescriptions but also as part of routine care. This process requires obtaining and verifying a comprehensive and accurate list of all medications currently in use, including drug names, dosages, frequency, and routes of administration [50]. This evaluation serves as the foundation of clinical medication review, requiring alignment of each drug with its indication and careful history taking to detect interactions or adverse reactions [51]. Regular assessments can aid in the early identification of medications that may contribute to the use of PIMs.

2.2.3 Prescribing habits

Physician prescribing habits represent a key contributor to inappropriate medication use in older adults. Long-standing clinical routines and reliance on established prescribing patterns may lead to the continuation of PIMs, even when safer or more effective alternatives exist. Such habits may be reinforced by familiarity with medications, peer learning, physicians' own beliefs, poor adaptability to change and inadequate acceptance of therapeutic alternatives, perceived patient expectations, or limited awareness of updated geriatric prescribing guidelines [52]. Incorporating geriatric pharmacology into continuing medical education to improve physicians' knowledge of geriatric prescribing may change their prescribing habits.

2.2.4 Fragmented care

Inadequate communication between prescribers, leading to unawareness of previously prescribed medications, may contribute to drug duplication, delayed identification of adverse events, and the initiation of prescribing cascades. The absence of effective communication among prescribers, amplified by insufficient documentation of therapeutic changes—including initiation, modification, and discontinuation, poses a significant risk to medication safety [53]. Given these considerations, effective communication of patients' health status with their physicians is essential, yet particularly challenging in older adults, owing to cognitive difficulties. This underscores the need for physicians to adopt a more deliberate approach in patient encounters and to enhance interprofessional consultation.

2.3 System-related factors

2.3.1 Insufficient comprehensive medication management programs

The management of chronic patients with comorbidities requires multidisciplinary teams that ensure patient-centered continuity of care, with active involvement of both the patient and their support network. The adoption of Comprehensive Medication Management (CMM) has been demonstrated to be an effective approach for the management of these conditions [54]. CMM is a patient-centered approach delivered by healthcare professionals that aims to optimize medication use, enhance safety and adherence, and improve overall health outcomes [55]. This model fosters collaborative engagement between patients and healthcare providers. Like other healthcare interventions, the implementation of CMM requires systematic data collection and timely reporting to inform clinical and population-level management. A consensus on appropriate quality and outcome metrics is necessary to evaluate and communicate the value of CMM services [56]. Considering all these factors, it is essential to use medication management programs to ensure that healthcare professionals have access to up-to-date health information.

2.3.2 Time constraints preventing medication reconciliation

Medication reconciliation is the process of establishing the most accurate list of all medications a patient is taking—including active ingredients, dosages, frequencies, and routes of administration—by comparing medical records with external sources, such as patient-provided lists or information from hospitals and other healthcare providers [57]. Medication reconciliation also involves a structured interview between the patient and the healthcare team to determine which prescription and over-the-counter medications are actually being taken [58]. Health systems must ensure that medical assistants have adequate time, resources, and communication tools to perform medication reconciliation effectively, while also optimizing the conditions under which this work is conducted. Time limitations during patient consultations are among the most commonly reported barriers, as clinicians often lack sufficient opportunity to perform comprehensive medication reviews and engage in discussions regarding deprescribing with their patients [59]. To address this challenge, healthcare systems should allocate sufficient consultation time and implement structured workflows that enable clinicians to perform comprehensive medication reviews and discuss deprescribing with patients effectively.

2.3.3 Insufficient communication between providers, pharmacies, and caregivers

Effective communication is essential not only among healthcare professionals but also between professionals and caregivers, particularly in patient populations requiring substantial support, such as older adults. Communication between pharmacists and other healthcare professionals can facilitate patient access to medication history. Improving communication between healthcare professionals and patients and their caregivers plays a key role in detecting PIM [60]. Healthcare professionals communicating with patients or caregivers both verbally and in writing can ensure a solid foundation for treatment [61]. This can vary depending on health literacy levels. Providing written communication to individuals with low health literacy is extremely important in presenting a healthy report to other healthcare professionals.

2.3.4 Financial barriers

Another system-related factor is the economic situation of the patients. Patients may choose to use medications that are not suitable for them because they are cheaper. Socioeconomic indicators, such as income, education, occupation, and neighborhood, have been reported to influence individuals' healthcare experiences. Populations with lower socioeconomic status are more likely to receive care of lower quality [62]. In populations with lower socioeconomic status, inadequate care coordination and substandard healthcare services may contribute to polypharmacy and the use of PIMs [63]. Low socioeconomic status may influence medication use in older adults through factors, such as inadequate prescriptions, reliance on older or generic drugs, and underutilization of appropriate medications [64, 65]. Government support can help mitigate the impact of low socioeconomic status on medication use, improving access to appropriate therapies and reducing the risk of polypharmacy and PIMs.

3. Consequences of inappropriate medication use

3.1 Adverse drug events

Medication selection is crucial in the elderly population because inappropriate prescribing can lead to ADEs. In older adults, ADEs are associated with increased emergency department visits, hospitalizations, healthcare costs, and higher morbidity and mortality rates [66, 67]. ADEs encompass harm directly attributable to medications—such as adverse drug reactions and overdoses—as well as harm associated with medication use, including dose reductions or discontinuations [68]. Although ADEs may arise from medication errors, the majority occur independently of such errors. Numerous studies have demonstrated that older adults experience higher rates of ADRs compared to younger individuals, with advancing age identified as a significant risk factor [69]. Age-related factors associated with an increased risk of ADRs in older adults include physiological age-related changes, multimorbidity, polypharmacy, frailty, and cognitive and sensory impairment [70–72]. Several criteria are available to assess the likelihood that an ADR is attributable to a specific drug, including the Naranjo Algorithm [73] and the Liverpool ADR Causality Assessment Tool [74]. Using this algorithm in geriatric patients, it can be determined whether adverse events occurring are drug related. When comparing drug classes among themselves in this population, the classes that cause the most adverse reactions are as follows: antipsychotics, anticoagulants, diuretics, analgesics, and anti-inflammatory [75, 76]. Adverse drug reactions of some drugs most used in geriatric populations are listed in **Table 1** [77–80].

These drugs, which are frequently used in elderly patients and cause adverse drug reactions, also carry the risk of being classified as PIM. Mitigating the risk of drug-induced adverse reactions necessitates the adoption of a comprehensive, systematic strategy. In certain instances, ADRs may be mitigated by dose reduction or, when appropriate, by discontinuation of the offending agent. Following the identification of a PIM, it is recommended to engage with the prescribing physician to reassess the clinical necessity of the medication and to consider its deprescription, where appropriate. Under professional healthcare, deprescribing entails reducing or discontinuing the use of inappropriate medications. The primary goal is to manage polypharmacy to reduce unnecessary or potentially harmful medication use and improve outcomes.

3.2 Increased hospitalizations

Patients exposed to PIM have been shown to have a higher risk of hospitalization compared to unexposed patients [81–83]. With growing evidence that exposure to

System	ADRs	Drug involved	Pharmacological group
Gastrointestinal	Gastrointestinal ulcer	Aspirin	Antithrombotic agents
		Clopidogrel	
		Warfarin	
	Constipation	Amlodipine	Antihypertensive
		Morphine	Opioid
		Tramadol	Opioid
		Verapamil	Antihypertensive
	Diarrhea	Lactulose	Laxative
		Metformin	Antidiabetic agent
Cardiovascular	Hypotension	Enalapril, Perindopril	Antihypertensive
	Edema	Amlodipine, Nifedipine	Antihypertensive
	Tachycardia	Salbutamol	Beta-2 agonist
		Theophylline	Phosphodiesterase enzyme inhibitor
	Bradycardia	Metoprolol	Antidiabetic agent
Endocrine and metabolic	Hypoglycemia	Insulin	Antidiabetic agent
	Hyperglycemia	Dexamethasone	Corticosteroid
	Hyperkalemia	Spironolactone	Diuretic
		Enalapril	Antihypertensive
Hematologic	Anemia	Pantoprazole	Proton pump inhibitor
		Levodopa	Anti-Parkinson agent
		Metformin	Antidiabetic agent
	Thrombocytopenia	Heparin	Anticoagulant
	Bleeding	Warfarin	Anticoagulant
Dermatologic	Hypersensitivity	Amoxicillin/clavulanate	Antibiotic
Neuromuscular and skeletal	Myalgia	Atorvastatin	Antilipemic agent
Others	Dry cough	Lisinopril	Antihypertensive
	Electrolyte and fluid balance conditions	Furosemide	Diuretic
		Valsartan	Antihypertensive
	Dizziness	Amitriptyline	Tricyclic antidepressant
		Olanzapine	Antipsychotic

Table 1.
Adverse drug reactions caused by certain medications in older adults.

PIMs elevates the risk of hospitalization, it is essential to delineate the risks linked to specific drug classes and individual agents. Thorough identification of high-risk medications is crucial to inform and guide clinical decision-making. High-risk medication classes associated with increased hospitalization include antithrombotics (anticoagulants and antiplatelets) [84], cardiovascular drugs (diuretics, angiotensin-converting enzyme inhibitors, beta-blockers) [84–86], nonsteroidal anti-inflammatory drugs

(NSAIDs) [87], antipsychotics [88], and hypoglycemics [89]. Identifying medication-related problems can prevent hospitalizations and other related health problems.

3.3 Fall and frailty

Frailty, reflecting cumulative age-related physiological decline, predisposes individuals to adverse drug events and greater medication-related harm. Frailty may arise from various factors, including sociodemographic conditions (e.g., poverty, social isolation, low education), psychological issues (e.g., depression), nutritional deficiencies (e.g., malnutrition), polypharmacy, chronic diseases and complications (e.g., inflammatory disorders, cancer, endocrine diseases, dementia), and physical inactivity. Regardless of its specific definition, frailty is a dynamic and multidimensional geriatric syndrome marked by fluctuating severity and multisystem impairment [90]. Fractures resulting from falls in the elderly can trigger a complex process. Falls impose a considerable burden on the healthcare system due to costly treatments required for injuries like hip fractures, including hospitalization and potential complications [91]. A recent study reported a stronger association between fall risk and the use of long-acting benzodiazepines, selective serotonin reuptake inhibitors, and serotonin-norepinephrine reuptake inhibitors [92]. According to the Beers Criteria, proton pump inhibitors (PPIs) are not recommended for use beyond 8 weeks because of their association with osteoporosis and increased fracture risk [9].

3.4 Increased healthcare costs

The use of PIMs contributes to increased healthcare expenditures, primarily through higher rates of hospitalizations, treatment of adverse drug events, prolonged disease management, and the added complexity of polypharmacy. An aging population is placing an increasing financial burden on healthcare systems through increased expenses, such as hospitalizations, long-term care, and chronic disease management [2]. One study reported that the direct costs of PIMs, encompassing both drug expenses and dispensing fees, amounted to $419 million [93]. Various initiatives that encourage appropriate prescribing and discontinuation have been proven to reduce PIM costs by 33% [94]. Therefore, identifying and correcting PIMs not only positively affects patient health but also provides a cost advantage.

4. Treatment management strategies

Appropriate treatment management strategies after PIM detection may require a multifaceted approach. This approach will be more effective, if it is implemented on a patient, healthcare system, and healthcare professional basis.

4.1 Clinical interventions

4.1.1 Medication review and reconciliation

Medication review is a vital process for evaluating a patient's pharmacotherapy and supporting appropriate deprescribing, warranting careful attention. Medication reviews can be conducted at varying levels—simple, intermediate, or advanced—depending on the type and source of available information, the degree of patient involvement, and the extent of multidisciplinary collaboration [95]. In this multidisciplinary process, pharmacists play a pivotal role in conducting medication reviews for older adults, applying a patient-centered approach that integrates both explicit and implicit criteria. This combined method has been shown to reduce the risk of ADEs and provide a more comprehensive assessment of overall medication management [96, 97]. Physicians may not have enough time to review medications with their patients due to time constraints during regular medical checkups. Therefore, pharmacists can turn this situation to their advantage. By meeting with the patient regularly, they thoroughly review medication dosages, side effects, pDDIs, route of administration, and timing of administration. They can also communicate with the physician to prevent potential PIMs. When conducting a comprehensive geriatric evaluation, physicians should also use criteria, such as Beers, TIME, and START-STOPP to determine the presence of PIM.

4.1.2 Deprescribing

Deprescribing studies highlight the crucial role of patient and family engagement in successfully discontinuing medications that cause actual or potential harm or offer minimal therapeutic benefit [98]. Multidisciplinary collaboration is essential in this process. Pharmaceutical care has been shown to enhance prescribing for older adults, particularly when the deprescribing process involves a multidisciplinary approach that integrates a clinical pharmacist [99]. Mitigating the risk of drug-induced adverse reactions necessitates the adoption of a comprehensive, systematic strategy. In certain instances, ADRs may be mitigated by dose reduction or, when appropriate, by discontinuation of the offending agent. Following the identification of a PIM, it is recommended to engage with the prescribing physician to reassess the clinical necessity of the medication and to consider its deprescription, where appropriate. Under professional healthcare, deprescribing entails reducing or discontinuing the use of inappropriate medications. The primary goal is to manage polypharmacy to reduce unnecessary or potentially harmful medication use and improve outcomes [100, 101]. The deprescribing process consists of five stages and is given in **Figure 1** [102].

To mitigate the burden of PIM, pharmaceutical care strategies—such as structured medication reviews and clinical decision support systems—should be incorporated into a comprehensive assessment of patients' clinical profiles, individual needs, and health priorities, thereby facilitating personalized prescribing and care planning.

4.1.3 Personalized prescribing

Individualized prescribing constitutes an important initiative in minimizing the use of PIMs. The use of clinical decision support systems is essential to optimize accuracy in personalized prescribing. Through these systems, patient data can be used to optimize the dosage of drugs according to their physiological systems. Integrating decision support tools with patient-specific data, such as renal function (creatinine clearance) and drug-metabolizing capacity (e.g., cytochrome P450 (CYP450) enzymes), offers significant potential for more tailored prescribing, advancing the practice of personalized medicine [103, 104]. Personalized medicine offers a promising approach to the growing challenge of polypharmacy in older adults, who often receive multiple medications for various conditions. By tailoring therapy to an individual's genetic profile, healthcare providers can reduce harmful drug interactions, enhance treatment efficacy, and ultimately improve the quality of care [2]. Selecting

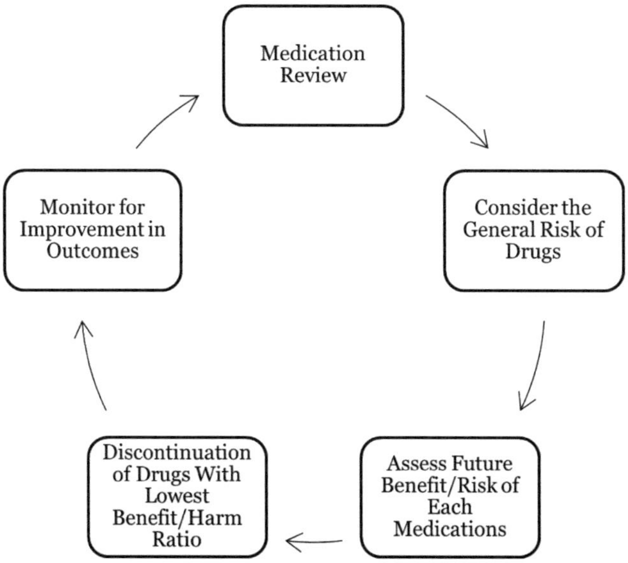

Figure 1.
Deprescribing process steps.

medications or adjusting dosages according to a patient's renal and hepatic function can help prevent future health complications. Likewise, considering the patient's pDDI profile when choosing therapy can promote optimal treatment outcomes.

4.1.4 Adherence support

In certain cases, PIMs may result from an improper medication use, which is directly influenced by patient adherence to treatment. Effective communication among healthcare providers is crucial for establishing a strong therapeutic partnership with patients and can enhance medication adherence [85]. Enhancing healthcare providers' communication skills in patient-centered pharmaceutical care should prioritize building rapport with older adults, which can improve treatment adherence [42]. Another approach is to reduce dosing frequency. For example, it has been reported that, on average, adherence decreases from approximately 80% in patients taking medication once daily to 50% in patients taking medication four times daily [105]. Through comprehensive geriatric assessment, physicians can gather detailed information on medication adherence from patients, family members, and caregivers, identify factors contributing to poor adherence, and implement interventions to prevent nonadherence [106, 107]. When appropriate, physicians, in collaboration with pharmacists, should consider simplifying medication regimens through single-dose packaging, reminder systems, or dosage form adjustments [108]. Following interventions to improve treatment adherence, reevaluation may be necessary to ensure ongoing consistency in the process.

4.2 System-level interventions

CMM represents a critical intervention to enhance both the safety and effectiveness of pharmacotherapy. Pharmacists are a potential resource to assist in the investigation of medications, so patients should review all information related to their pharmaceutical care and resolve any suspicions about PIM by contacting the patient's physician immediately [109]. Pharmacist-led medication reviews have been identified as a key strategy in addressing medication-related problems, including PIMs, regimen complexity, and discrepancies in prescriptions. Evidence indicates that inappropriate prescribing among older adults is significantly reduced when pharmacists and other healthcare professionals, including physicians, collaborate within multidisciplinary teams across healthcare sectors [110]. Notably, the involvement of clinical pharmacists in hospital discharge care transitions—through activities such as medication reconciliation, review, counseling, and post-discharge follow-up—has been shown to significantly reduce hospital readmissions and post-discharge visits [111]. Interprofessional medication management has demonstrated effectiveness in enhancing the quality of outpatient pharmacotherapy for polypharmacy, multimorbid older adults, while also reducing the incidence of medication-related problems [112]. Effective implementation of interprofessional medication management requires collaborative interventions, such as medication reconciliation, patient and healthcare professional education, integration of computerized decision support tools, and the joint application of geriatric-specific criteria [113, 114]. Computerized decision support tools provide access to a wide range of pharmaceutical care services, including the identification of pDDIs, monitoring of drug-related adverse effects and biochemical parameters, evaluation of high medication use, and patient counseling on appropriate medication practices. Multifaceted pharmaceutical interventions—incorporating medication evaluation, motivational interviewing, and post-discharge follow-up—have been shown to reduce hospital readmission rates both in the short- and long term among patients hospitalized for polypharmacy [115, 116]. If all these system-related factors mentioned are implemented together, the existence of PIM will largely disappear.

4.3 Patient and caregiver engagement

Another intervention is to raise awareness, encourage, and provide education about the treatment provided to the patient or caregiver. The literature consistently highlights patient education as a crucial strategy for improving medication adherence [117]. A considerable portion of orally communicated information may be forgotten by patients; therefore, providing written materials is essential to reinforce key messages, promote safe medication use, improve treatment adherence, and enhance patient satisfaction with care [117, 118]. Moreover, combining visual cues with verbal instructions has been shown to enhance patients' recall compared to verbal instructions alone. Encouraging patients and caregivers to report drug-related adverse events enhances the quality of drug safety data within health systems and facilitates early detection of potential risks. Accordingly, strategies including patient education, accessible reporting mechanisms, and supportive engagement from healthcare professionals are essential to promote greater participation [119]. It has also been emphasized that caregivers play a vital role in ensuring prescriptions are taken on time and in monitoring patients for potential side effects [120]. Additionally, caregivers assist with the administration of prescribed treatments and may coordinate rehabilitative interventions, including speech and physical therapy [121].

5. Conclusion

Reducing PIM requires a multifaceted approach that includes identifying patients potentially at risk for PIM, comprehensive medication review, deprescribing, assessing patient compliance, education for healthcare providers and patients, improvements in the work environment, and integration of computer-aided technologies to detect inappropriate medications. Therefore, strengthening interdisciplinary collaboration remains a cornerstone for minimizing PIM use and improving overall quality of care in older adults. In addition, future research focusing on the long-term outcomes of such interventions will provide valuable insights for optimizing geriatric pharmacotherapy.

Acknowledgements

This study was conducted during the health problems experienced by one of the authors, and we would like to express our gratitude to the authors who contributed to the study for their deep friendship, with which we believe they will see many more days together, despite all the difficulties.

Conflict of interest

The authors declare no conflict of interest.

Author details

Ahmet Çakır[1*] and Hasan Memiş[2]

1 Department of Clinical Pharmacy, Faculty of Pharmacy, Inonu University, Malatya, Türkiye

2 Department of Clinical Pharmacy, University of Health Sciences Konya Beyhekim Training and Research Hospital, Konya, Türkiye

*Address all correspondence to: eczahmetcakir@hotmail.com

References

[1] McHugh D, Gil J. Senescence and aging: Causes, consequences, and therapeutic avenues. The Journal of Cell Biology. 2018;**217**(1):65-77. DOI: 10.1083/jcb.201708092

[2] Shreya D, Fish PN, Du D. Navigating the future of elderly healthcare: A comprehensive analysis of aging populations and mortality trends using National Inpatient Sample (NIS) data (2010-2024). Cureus. 2025;**17**(3):e80442. DOI: 10.7759/cureus.80442

[3] Lavan AH, Gallagher P. Predicting risk of adverse drug reactions in older adults. Therapeutic Advances in Drug Safety. 2016;**7**(1):11-22. DOI: 10.1177/2042098615615472

[4] Tian F, Chen Z, Zeng Y, Feng Q, Chen X. Prevalence of use of potentially inappropriate medications among older adults worldwide: A systematic review and meta-analysis. JAMA Network Open. 2023;**6**(8):e2326910. DOI: 10.1001/jamanetworkopen.2023.26910

[5] Rambhade S, Chakarborty A, Shrivastava A, Patil UK, Rambhade A. A survey on polypharmacy and use of inappropriate medications. Toxicology International. 2012;**19**(1):68-73. DOI: 10.4103/0971-6580.94506

[6] Curtin D, Gallagher PF, O'Mahony D. Explicit criteria as clinical tools to minimize inappropriate medication use and its consequences. Therapeutic Advances in Drug Safety. 2019;**10**:2042098619829431. DOI: 10.1177/2042098619829431

[7] Maher RL, Hanlon J, Hajjar ER. Clinical consequences of polypharmacy in elderly. Expert Opinion on Drug Safety. 2014;**13**(1):57-65. DOI: 10.1517/14740338.2013.827660

[8] Nothelle SK, Sharma R, Oakes A, Jackson M, Segal JB. Factors associated with potentially inappropriate medication use in community-dwelling older adults in the United States: A systematic review. The International Journal of Pharmacy Practice. 2019;**27**(5):408-423. DOI: 10.1111/ijpp.12541

[9] American Geriatrics Society Beers Criteria Update Expert Panel. American Geriatrics Society 2023 updated AGS Beers Criteria® for potentially inappropriate medication use in older adults. Journal of the American Geriatrics Society. 2023;**71**(7):2052-2081. DOI: 10.1111/jgs.18372

[10] Bahat G, Ilhan B, Erdogan T, Halil M, Savas S, Ulger Z, et al. Turkish inappropriate medication use in the elderly (TIME) criteria to improve prescribing in older adults: TIME-to-STOP/TIME-to-START. European Geriatric Medicine. 2020;**11**(3):491-498. DOI: 10.1007/s41999-020-00297-z

[11] Akyön ŞH, Sılay K, Thürmann PA. Tools to reduce inappropriate drug use in geriatric patients: PRISCUS 2.0 list updates. Archives of Gerontology and Geriatrics Plus. 2024;**1**(4):100052. DOI: 10.1016/j.aggp.2024.100052

[12] O'Mahony D, Cherubini A, Guiteras AR, Denkinger M, Beuscart JB, Onder G, et al. STOPP/START criteria for potentially inappropriate prescribing in older people: Version 3. European Geriatric Medicine. 2023;**14**(4):625-632. DOI: 10.1007/s41999-023-00777-y

[13] Pazan F, Weiss C, Wehling M. The EURO-FORTA (Fit fOR The Aged) list version 2: Consensus validation of a clinical tool for improved pharmacotherapy in older adults.

Drugs & Aging. 2023;**40**(5):417-426. DOI: 10.1007/s40266-023-01024-6

[14] Huang Y, Zhang L, Huang X, Liu K, Yu Y, Xiao J. Potentially inappropriate medications in Chinese community-dwelling older adults. Int. Journal of Clinical Pharmacology. 2020;**42**(2):598-603. DOI: 10.1007/s11096-020-00980-y

[15] Renom-Guiteras A, Meyer G, Thürmann PA. The EU(7)-PIM list: A list of potentially inappropriate medications for older people consented by experts from seven European countries. European Journal of Clinical Pharmacology. 2015;**71**(7):861-875. DOI: 10.1007/s00228-015-1860-9

[16] Pazan F, Wehling M. Polypharmacy in older adults: A narrative review of definitions, epidemiology and consequences. European Geriatric Medicine. 2021;**12**(3):443-452. DOI: 10.1007/s41999-021-00479-3

[17] Stuhec M, Zorjan K. Clinical pharmacist interventions in ambulatory psychogeriatric patients with excessive polypharmacy. Scientific Reports. 2022;**12**(1):11387. DOI: 10.1038/s41598-022-15657-x

[18] Wastesson JW, Morin L, Tan ECK, Johnell K. An update on the clinical consequences of polypharmacy in older adults: A narrative review. Expert Opinion on Drug Safety. 2018;**17**(12):1185-1196. DOI: 10.1080/14740338.2018.1546841

[19] Dovjak P. Polypharmacy in elderly people. Wiener Medizinische Wochenschrift (1946). 2022;**172**(5-6):109-113. DOI: 10.1007/s10354-021-00903-0

[20] Kim J, Parish AL. Polypharmacy and medication management in older adults. The Nursing Clinics of North America. 2017;**52**(3):457-468. DOI: 10.1016/j.cnur.2017.04.007

[21] Zazzara MB, Palmer K, Vetrano DL, Carfì A, Onder G. Adverse drug reactions in older adults: A narrative review of the literature. European Geriatric Medicine. 2021;**12**(3):463-473. DOI: 10.1007/s41999-021-00481-9

[22] Jiang H, Lin Y, Ren W, Lu L, Tan X, Lv X, et al. Potential inappropriate medications and drug-drug interactions in adverse drug reactions in the elderly: A retrospective study in a pharmacovigilance database. Frontiers in Pharmacology. 2025;**16**:1546012. DOI: 10.3389/fphar.2025.1546012

[23] Endalifer BL, Kassa MT, Ejigu YW, Ambaye AS. Polypharmacy, drug-drug interactions, and potentially inappropriate medications among older adults: A cross-sectional study in Northeast Ethiopia. Frontiers in Public Health. 2025;**13**:1525079. DOI: 10.3389/fpubh.2025.1525079

[24] Laberge M, Sirois C, Lunghi C, Gaudreault M, Nakamura Y, Bolduc C, et al. Economic evaluations of interventions to optimize medication use in older adults with polypharmacy and multimorbidity: A systematic review. Clinical Interventions in Aging. 2021;**16**:767-779. DOI: 10.2147/cia.S304074

[25] Xu X, Mishra GD, Jones M. Evidence on multimorbidity from definition to intervention: An overview of systematic reviews. Ageing Research Reviews. 2017;**37**:53-68. DOI: 10.1016/j.arr.2017.05.003

[26] Yarnall AJ, Sayer AA, Clegg A, Rockwood K, Parker S, Hindle JV. New horizons in multimorbidity in older adults. Age and Ageing. 2017;**46**(6):882-888. DOI: 10.1093/ageing/afx150

[27] Borrie M, Cooper T, Basu M, Kay K, Prorok JC, Seitz D. Ontario geriatric specialist physician resources 2018. Canadian Geriatrics Journal. 2020;**23**(3):219-227. DOI: 10.5770/cgj.23.448

[28] Nguyen H, Manolova G, Daskalopoulou C, Vitoratou S, Prince M, Prina AM. Prevalence of multimorbidity in community settings: A systematic review and meta-analysis of observational studies. Journal of Comorbidity. 2019;**9**:2235042x19870934. DOI: 10.1177/2235042x19870934

[29] Jaul E, Barron J. Age-related diseases and clinical and public health implications for the 85 years old and over population. Frontiers in Public Health. 2017;**5**:335. DOI: 10.3389/fpubh.2017.00335

[30] Gnjidic D, Husband A, Todd A. Challenges and innovations of delivering medicines to older adults. Advanced Drug Delivery Reviews. 2018;**135**:97-105. DOI: 10.1016/j.addr.2018.08.003

[31] Kojima T, Mizokami F, Akishita M. Geriatric management of older patients with multimorbidity. Geriatrics & Gerontology International. 2020;**20**(12): 1105-1111. DOI: 10.1111/ggi.14065

[32] Aalami OO, Fang TD, Song HM, Nacamuli RP. Physiological features of aging persons. Archives of Surgery. 2003;**138**(10):1068-1076. DOI: 10.1001/archsurg.138.10.1068

[33] Mangoni AA, Jackson SH. Age-related changes in pharmacokinetics and pharmacodynamics: Basic principles and practical applications. British Journal of Clinical Pharmacology. 2004;**57**(1):6-14. DOI: 10.1046/j.1365-2125.2003.02007.x

[34] Moore AR, O'Keeffe ST. Drug-induced cognitive impairment in the elderly. Drugs & Aging. 1999;**15**(1):15-28. DOI: 10.2165/00002512-199915010-00002

[35] Lam RW, Kennedy SH, McLntyre RS, Khullar A. Cognitive dysfunction in major depressive disorder: Effects on psychosocial functioning and implications for treatment. Canadian Journal of Psychiatry. 2014;**59**(12):649-654. DOI: 10.1177/070674371405901206

[36] Majmundar MK, Hayward MD. Future Directions for the Demography of Aging: Proceedings of a Workshop. Washington, DC: National Academies Press (US); 2018. DOI: 10.17226/25064

[37] Reimers A, Odin P, Ljung H. Drug-induced cognitive impairment. Drug Safety. 2025;**48**(4):339-361. DOI: 10.1007/s40264-024-01506-5

[38] World Health Organization. The Role of the Pharmacist in Self-Care and Self-Medication: Report of the 4th WHO Consultative Group on the Role of the Pharmacist, The Hague, The Netherlands, 26-28 August 1998. Geneva, The Netherlands: Department of Essential Drugs and Other Medicines, World Health Organization; 1998

[39] Ruiz ME. Risks of self-medication practices. Current Drug Safety. 2010;**5**(4):315-323. DOI: 10.2174/157488610792245966

[40] Chapman SCE, Chan AHY. Medication nonadherence—Definition, measurement, prevalence, and causes: Reflecting on the past 20 years and looking forwards. Frontiers in Pharmacology. 2025;**16**:1465059. DOI: 10.3389/fphar.2025.1465059

[41] Kim S, Bennett K, Wallace E, Fahey T, Cahir C. Measuring medication adherence in older community-dwelling patients with multimorbidity. European

Journal of Clinical Pharmacology. 2018;**74**(3):357-364. DOI: 10.1007/s00228-017-2388-y

[42] Jin H, Kim Y, Rhie SJ. Factors affecting medication adherence in elderly people. Patient Preference and Adherence. 2016;**10**:2117-2125. DOI: 10.2147/ppa.S118121

[43] Schiff GD, Fung S, Speroff T, McNutt RA. Decompensated heart failure: Symptoms, patterns of onset, and contributing factors. The American Journal of Medicine. 2003;**114**(8):625-630. DOI: 10.1016/s0002-9343(03)00132-3

[44] Sokol MC, McGuigan KA, Verbrugge RR, Epstein RS. Impact of medication adherence on hospitalization risk and healthcare cost. Medical Care. 2005;**43**(6):521-530. DOI: 10.1097/01.mlr.0000163641.86870.af

[45] Morisky DE, Ang A, Krousel-Wood M, Ward HJ. Predictive validity of a medication adherence measure in an outpatient setting. Journal of Clinical Hypertension (Greenwich, Conn.). 2008;**10**(5):348-354. DOI: 10.1111/j.1751-7176.2008.07572.x

[46] Rochon PA, Gurwitz JH. The prescribing cascade revisited. Lancet. 2017;**389**(10081):1778-1780. DOI: 10.1016/s0140-6736(17)31188-1

[47] Savage RD, Visentin JD, Bronskill SE, Wang X, Gruneir A, Giannakeas V, et al. Evaluation of a common prescribing cascade of calcium channel blockers and diuretics in older adults with hypertension. JAMA Internal Medicine. 2020;**180**(5):643-651. DOI: 10.1001/jamainternmed.2019.7087

[48] Vouri SM, Jiang X, Manini TM, Solberg LM, Pepine C, Malone DC, et al. Magnitude of and characteristics associated with the treatment of calcium channel blocker-induced lower-extremity edema with loop diuretics. JAMA Network Open. 2019;**2**(12):e1918425. DOI: 10.1001/jamanetworkopen.2019.18425

[49] Griese-Mammen N, Hersberger KE, Messerli M, Leikola S, Horvat N, van Mil JWF, et al. PCNE definition of medication review: Reaching agreement. International Journal of Clinical Pharmacy. 2018;**40**(5):1199-1208. DOI: 10.1007/s11096-018-0696-7

[50] Jarrett T, Cochran J, Baus A. Applying the medications at transitions and clinical handoffs toolkit in a rural primary care clinic: Implications for nursing, patients, and caregivers. Journal of Nursing Care Quality. 2020;**35**(3):233-239. DOI: 10.1097/ncq.0000000000000454

[51] Somers A, Mallet L, van der Cammen T, Robays H, Petrovic M. Applicability of an adapted medication appropriateness index for detection of drug-related problems in geriatric inpatients. The American Journal of Geriatric Pharmacotherapy. 2012;**10**(2):101-109. DOI: 10.1016/j.amjopharm.2012.01.003

[52] Lau S, Lun P, Ang W, Tan KT, Ding YY. Barriers to effective prescribing in older adults: Applying the theoretical domains framework in the ambulatory setting—A scoping review. BMC Geriatrics. 2020;**20**(1):459. DOI: 10.1186/s12877-020-01766-7

[53] Cullinan S, Raae Hansen C, Byrne S, O'Mahony D, Kearney P, Sahm L. Challenges of deprescribing in the multimorbid patient. European Journal of Hospital Pharmacy. 2017;**24**(1):43-46. DOI: 10.1136/ejhpharm-2016-000921

[54] McFarland MS, Buck ML, Crannage E, Armistead LT, Ourth H,

Finks SW, et al. Assessing the impact of comprehensive medication management on achievement of the quadruple aim. The American Journal of Medicine. 2021;**134**(4):456-461. DOI: 10.1016/j.amjmed.2020.12.008

[55] Pestka D, Sorge L, Mendkoff J, Frail C, Funk K, Sorensen T, et al. Assessing the state of comprehensive medication management in a sample of primary care clinics. Innovations in Pharmacy. 2019;**10**(1):1-9. DOI: 10.24926/iip.v10i1.1611

[56] Haas CE, Kliethermes MA, Armistead LT, Beavers C, Schumacher C, Smith L, et al. Comprehensive medication management: Review and recommendations for quality measures. Journal of the American College of Clinical Pharmacy. 2023;**6**(4):404-415. DOI: 10.1002/jac5.1767

[57] Rattray D, Whitner VerVaet J, Lisenby K. Medication Reconciliation Guidance Document for Pharmacists. American Health-System Pharmacists Section Advisory Group on Medication Management Services; 2018

[58] Commission J. Ambulatory Health Care National Patient Safety Goals. 2012

[59] Sutanto H. Tackling polypharmacy in geriatric patients: Is increasing physicians' awareness adequate? Archives of Gerontology and Geriatrics Plus. 2025;**2**(3):100185. DOI: 10.1016/j.aggp.2025.100185

[60] Copley DM, Manias E, Watkins V, Hutchinson AM. Communication processes related to decision-making in medication management between healthcare providers, older people and their carers: A systematic review. Health Expectations. 2025;**28**(2):e70252. DOI: 10.1111/hex.70252

[61] Sharkiya SH. Quality communication can improve patient-centred health outcomes among older patients: A rapid review. BMC Health Services Research. 2023;**23**(1):886. DOI: 10.1186/s12913-023-09869-8

[62] Asch SM, Kerr EA, Keesey J, Adams JL, Setodji CM, Malik S, et al. Who is at greatest risk for receiving poor-quality health care? The New England Journal of Medicine. 2006;**354**(11):1147-1156. DOI: 10.1056/NEJMsa044464

[63] Toivo T, Dimitrow M, Puustinen J, Savela E, Pelkonen K, Kiuru V, et al. Coordinating resources for prospective medication risk management of older home care clients in primary care: Procedure development and RCT study design for demonstrating its effectiveness. BMC Geriatrics. 2018;**18**(1):74. DOI: 10.1186/s12877-018-0737-z

[64] Odubanjo E, Bennett K, Feely J. Influence of socioeconomic status on the quality of prescribing in the elderly—A population based study. British Journal of Clinical Pharmacology. 2004;**58**(5):496-502. DOI: 10.1111/j.1365-2125.2004.02179.x

[65] Mamdani MM, Tu K, Austin PC, Alter DA. Influence of socioeconomic status on drug selection for the elderly in Canada. The Annals of Pharmacotherapy. 2002;**36**(5):804-808. DOI: 10.1345/aph.1A044

[66] O'Mahony D, Gallagher PF. Inappropriate prescribing in the older population: Need for new criteria. Age and Ageing. 2008;**37**(2):138-141. DOI: 10.1093/ageing/afm189

[67] Hartholt KA, van Beeck EF, Polinder S, van der Velde N, van Lieshout EM, Panneman MJ, et al. Societal consequences of falls in the older

population: Injuries, healthcare costs, and long-term reduced quality of life. The Journal of Trauma. 2011;**71**(3):748-753. DOI: 10.1097/TA.0b013e3181f6f5e5

[68] Nebeker JR, Barach P, Samore MH. Clarifying adverse drug events: A clinician's guide to terminology, documentation, and reporting. Annals of Internal Medicine. 2004;**140**(10):795-801. DOI: 10.7326/0003-4819-140-10-200405180-00009

[69] Patel NS, Patel TK, Patel PB, Naik VN, Tripathi CB. Hospitalizations due to preventable adverse reactions-a systematic review. European Journal of Clinical Pharmacology. 2017;**73**(4):385-398. DOI: 10.1007/s00228-016-2170-6

[70] Calderón-Larrañaga A, Vetrano DL, Onder G, Gimeno-Feliu LA, Coscollar-Santaliestra C, Carfí A, et al. Assessing and measuring chronic multimorbidity in the older population: A proposal for its operationalization. The Journals of Gerontology. Series A, Biological Sciences and Medical Sciences. 2017;**72**(10):1417-1423. DOI: 10.1093/gerona/glw233

[71] Moriarty F, Hardy C, Bennett K, Smith SM, Fahey T. Trends and interaction of polypharmacy and potentially inappropriate prescribing in primary care over 15 years in Ireland: A repeated cross-sectional study. BMJ Open. 2015;**5**(9):e008656. DOI: 10.1136/bmjopen-2015-008656

[72] Muhlack DC, Hoppe LK, Stock C, Haefeli WE, Brenner H, Schöttker B. The associations of geriatric syndromes and other patient characteristics with the current and future use of potentially inappropriate medications in a large cohort study. European Journal of Clinical Pharmacology. 2018;**74**(12):1633-1644. DOI: 10.1007/s00228-018-2534-1

[73] Naranjo CA, Busto U, Sellers EM, Sandor P, Ruiz I, Roberts EA, et al. A method for estimating the probability of adverse drug reactions. Clinical Pharmacology and Therapeutics. 1981;**30**(2):239-245. DOI: 10.1038/clpt.1981.154

[74] Gallagher RM, Kirkham JJ, Mason JR, Bird KA, Williamson PR, Nunn AJ, et al. Development and inter-rater reliability of the Liverpool adverse drug reaction causality assessment tool. PLoS ONE. 2011;**6**(12):e28096. DOI: 10.1371/journal.pone.0028096

[75] Davies EA, O'Mahony MS. Adverse drug reactions in special populations—The elderly. British Journal of Clinical Pharmacology. 2015;**80**(4):796-807. DOI: 10.1111/bcp.12596

[76] Woo SD, Yoon J, Doo GE, Park Y, Lee Y, Lee SH, et al. Common causes and characteristics of adverse drug reactions in older adults: A retrospective study. BMC. Pharmacology & Toxicology. 2020;**21**(1):87. DOI: 10.1186/s40360-020-00464-9

[77] Yadesa TM, Kitutu FE, Tamukong R, Alele PE. Prevalence, incidence, and characteristics of adverse drug reactions among older adults hospitalized at Mbarara regional referral hospital, Uganda: A prospective cohort study. Clinical Interventions in Aging. 2021;**16**:1705-1721. DOI: 10.2147/cia.S332251

[78] Dagnew SB, Moges TA, Ayele TM, Wondm SA, Yazie TS, Dagnew FN. Adverse drug reactions and its associated factors among geriatric hospitalized patients at selected comprehensive specialized hospitals of the Amhara region, Ethiopia: A multicenter prospective cohort study. BMC Geriatrics. 2024;**24**(1):955. DOI: 10.1186/s12877-024-05515-y

[79] Cahir C, Curran C, Walsh C, Hickey A, Brannigan R, Kirke C, et al. Adverse drug reactions in an ageing PopulaTion (ADAPT) study: Prevalence and risk factors associated with adverse drug reaction-related hospital admissions in older patients. Frontiers in Pharmacology. 2022;**13**:1029067. DOI: 10.3389/fphar.2022.1029067

[80] Gray SL, Sager M, Lestico MR, Jalaluddin M. Adverse drug events in hospitalized elderly. The Journals of Gerontology. Series A, Biological Sciences and Medical Sciences. 1998;**53**(1):M59-M63. DOI: 10.1093/gerona/53a.1.m59

[81] Brown JD, Hutchison LC, Li C, Painter JT, Martin BC. Predictive validity of the beers and screening tool of older persons' potentially inappropriate prescriptions (STOPP) criteria to detect adverse drug events, hospitalizations, and emergency department visits in the United States. Journal of the American Geriatrics Society. 2016;**64**(1):22-30. DOI: 10.1111/jgs.13884

[82] Reich O, Rosemann T, Rapold R, Blozik E, Senn O. Potentially inappropriate medication use in older patients in Swiss managed care plans: Prevalence, determinants and association with hospitalization. PLoS ONE. 2014;**9**(8):e105425. DOI: 10.1371/journal.pone.0105425

[83] Endres HG, Kaufmann-Kolle P, Steeb V, Bauer E, Böttner C, Thürmann P. Association between potentially inappropriate medication (PIM) use and risk of hospitalization in older adults: An observational study based on routine data comparing PIM use with use of PIM alternatives. PLoS ONE. 2016;**11**(2):e0146811. DOI: 10.1371/journal.pone.0146811

[84] Pedrós C, Quintana B, Rebolledo M, Porta N, Vallano A, Arnau JM. Prevalence, risk factors and main features of adverse drug reactions leading to hospital admission. European Journal of Clinical Pharmacology. 2014;**70**(3):361-367. DOI: 10.1007/s00228-013-1630-5

[85] Conforti A, Costantini D, Zanetti F, Moretti U, Grezzana M, Leone R. Adverse drug reactions in older patients: An Italian observational prospective hospital study. Drug, Healthcare and Patient Safety. 2012;**4**:75-80. DOI: 10.2147/dhps.S29287

[86] Ahern F, Sahm LJ, Lynch D, McCarthy S. Determining the frequency and preventability of adverse drug reaction-related admissions to an Irish University Hospital: A cross-sectional study. Emergency Medicine Journal. 2014;**31**(1):24-29. DOI: 10.1136/emermed-2012-201945

[87] Pirmohamed M, James S, Meakin S, Green C, Scott AK, Walley TJ, et al. Adverse drug reactions as cause of admission to hospital: Prospective analysis of 18 820 patients. BMJ. 2004;**329**(7456):15-19. DOI: 10.1136/bmj.329.7456.15

[88] Onder G, Pedone C, Landi F, Cesari M, Della Vedova C, Bernabei R, et al. Adverse drug reactions as cause of hospital admissions: Results from the Italian Group of Pharmacoepidemiology in the Elderly (GIFA). Journal of the American Geriatrics Society. 2002;**50**(12):1962-1968. DOI: 10.1046/j.1532-5415.2002.50607.x

[89] Olivier P, Bertrand L, Tubery M, Lauque D, Montastruc JL, Lapeyre-Mestre M. Hospitalizations because of adverse drug reactions in elderly patients admitted through the emergency department: A prospective survey. Drugs & Aging. 2009;**26**(6):475-482. DOI:10.2165/00002512-200926060-00004

[90] Di Ciaula A, Portincasa P. The environment as a determinant of successful aging or frailty. Mechanisms of Ageing and Development. 2020;**188**:111244. DOI: 10.1016/j.mad.2020.111244

[91] Dykes PC, Curtin-Bowen M, Lipsitz S, Franz C, Adelman J, Adkison L, et al. Cost of inpatient falls and cost-benefit analysis of implementation of an evidence-based fall prevention program. JAMA Health Forum. 2023;**4**(1):e225125. DOI: 10.1001/jamahealthforum.2022.5125

[92] Érszegi A, Csupor D, Bodó G, Engi Z, Bahar MA, Matuz M, et al. High rate of potentially inappropriate medication use in older people: A case-control study. Geroscience. 2024;**46**(5):5217-5233. DOI: 10.1007/s11357-024-01274-1

[93] Morgan SG, Hunt J, Rioux J, Proulx J, Weymann D, Tannenbaum C. Frequency and cost of potentially inappropriate prescribing for older adults: A cross-sectional study. CMAJ Open. 2016;**4**(2):E346-E351. DOI: 10.9778/cmajo.20150131

[94] Huon JF, Sanyal C, Gagnon CL, Turner JP, Khuong NB, Bortolussi-Courval É, et al. The cost of potentially inappropriate medications for older adults in Canada: A comparative cross-sectional study. Journal of the American Geriatrics Society. 2024;**72**(11):3530-3540. DOI: 10.1111/jgs.19164

[95] Spinewine A, Fialová D, Byrne S. The role of the pharmacist in optimizing pharmacotherapy in older people. Drugs & Aging. 2012;**29**(6):495-510. DOI: 10.2165/11631720-000000000-00000

[96] Petrovic M, van der Cammen T, Onder G. Adverse drug reactions in older people: Detection and prevention. Drugs & Aging. 2012;**29**(6):453-462. DOI: 10.2165/11631760-000000000-00000

[97] Hill-Taylor B, Sketris I, Hayden J, Byrne S, O'Sullivan D, Christie R. Application of the STOPP/START criteria: A systematic review of the prevalence of potentially inappropriate prescribing in older adults, and evidence of clinical, humanistic and economic impact. Journal of Clinical Pharmacy and Therapeutics. 2013;**38**(5):360-372. DOI: 10.1111/jcpt.12059

[98] Green AR, Aschmann H, Boyd CM, Schoenborn N. Assessment of patient-preferred language to achieve goal-aligned deprescribing in older adults. JAMA Network Open. 2021;**4**(4):e212633. DOI: 10.1001/jamanetworkopen.2021.2633

[99] Rankin A, Cadogan CA, Patterson SM, Kerse N, Cardwell CR, Bradley MC, et al. Interventions to improve the appropriate use of polypharmacy for older people. Cochrane Database of Systematic Reviews. 2018;**9**(9):Cd008165. DOI: 10.1002/14651858.CD008165.pub4

[100] Farrell B, Tsang C, Raman-Wilms L, Irving H, Conklin J, Pottie K. What are priorities for deprescribing for elderly patients? Capturing the voice of practitioners: A modified delphi process. PLoS ONE. 2015;**10**(4):e0122246. DOI: 10.1371/journal.pone.0122246

[101] Reeve E, Gnjidic D, Long J, Hilmer S. A systematic review of the emerging definition of 'deprescribing' with network analysis: Implications for future research and clinical practice. British Journal of Clinical Pharmacology. 2015;**80**(6):1254-1268. DOI: 10.1111/bcp.12732

[102] Scott IA, Hilmer SN, Reeve E, Potter K, Le Couteur D, Rigby D, et al.

Reducing inappropriate polypharmacy: The process of deprescribing. JAMA Internal Medicine. 2015;**175**(5):827-834. DOI: 10.1001/jamainternmed.2015.0324

[103] Brixner D, Biltaji E, Bress A, Unni S, Ye X, Mamiya T, et al. The effect of pharmacogenetic profiling with a clinical decision support tool on healthcare resource utilization and estimated costs in the elderly exposed to polypharmacy. Journal of Medical Economics. 2016;**19**(3):213-228. DOI: 10.3111/13696998.2015.1110160

[104] Elliott LS, Henderson JC, Neradilek MB, Moyer NA, Ashcraft KC, Thirumaran RK. Clinical impact of pharmacogenetic profiling with a clinical decision support tool in polypharmacy home health patients: A prospective pilot randomized controlled trial. PLoS ONE. 2017;**12**(2):e0170905. DOI: 10.1371/journal.pone.0170905

[105] Claxton AJ, Cramer J, Pierce C. A systematic review of the associations between dose regimens and medication compliance. Clinical Therapeutics. 2001;**23**(8):1296-1310. DOI: 10.1016/s0149-2918(01)80109-0

[106] Haynes RB, Ackloo E, Sahota N, McDonald HP, Yao X. Interventions for enhancing medication adherence. Cochrane Database of Systematic Reviews. 2008;(2):Cd000011. DOI: 10.1002/14651858.CD000011.pub3

[107] Kripalani S, Yao X, Haynes RB. Interventions to enhance medication adherence in chronic medical conditions: A systematic review. Archives of Internal Medicine. 2007;**167**(6):540-550. DOI: 10.1001/archinte.167.6.540

[108] Conn VS, Hafdahl AR, Cooper PS, Ruppar TM, Mehr DR, Russell CL. Interventions to improve medication adherence among older adults: Meta-analysis of adherence outcomes among randomized controlled trials. The Gerontologist. 2009;**49**(4):447-462. DOI: 10.1093/geront/gnp037

[109] Krska J, Cromarty JA, Arris F, Jamieson D, Hansford D, Duffus PR, et al. Pharmacist-led medication review in patients over 65: A randomized, controlled trial in primary care. Age and Ageing. 2001;**30**(3):205-211. DOI: 10.1093/ageing/30.3.205

[110] Gillespie U, Alassaad A, Hammarlund-Udenaes M, Mörlin C, Henrohn D, Bertilsson M, et al. Effects of pharmacists' interventions on appropriateness of prescribing and evaluation of the instruments' (MAI, STOPP and STARTs') ability to predict hospitalization--analyses from a randomized controlled trial. PLoS ONE. 2013;**8**(5):e62401. DOI: 10.1371/journal.pone.0062401

[111] Van der Linden L, Hias J, Walgraeve K, Flamaing J, Tournoy J, Spriet I. Clinical pharmacy services in older inpatients: An evidence-based review. Drugs & Aging. 2020;**37**(3):161-174. DOI: 10.1007/s40266-019-00733-1

[112] Köberlein-Neu J, Mennemann H, Hamacher S, Waltering I, Jaehde U, Schaffert C, et al. Interprofessional medication management in patients with multiple morbidities. Deutsches Ärzteblatt International. 2016;**113**(44):741-748. DOI: 10.3238/arztebl.2016.0741

[113] Dautzenberg L, Bretagne L, Koek HL, Tsokani S, Zevgiti S, Rodondi N, et al. Medication review interventions to reduce hospital readmissions in older people. Journal of the American Geriatrics Society. 2021;**69**(6):1646-1658. DOI: 10.1111/jgs.17041

[114] Avorn J, Soumerai SB, Everitt DE, Ross-Degnan D, Beers MH, Sherman D, et al. A randomized trial of a program to reduce the use of psychoactive drugs in nursing homes. The New England Journal of Medicine. 1992;**327**(3):168-173. DOI: 10.1056/nejm199207163270306

[115] Ravn-Nielsen LV, Duckert ML, Lund ML, Henriksen JP, Nielsen ML, Eriksen CS, et al. Effect of an in-hospital multifaceted clinical pharmacist intervention on the risk of readmission: A randomized clinical trial. JAMA Internal Medicine. 2018;**178**(3):375-382. DOI: 10.1001/jamainternmed.2017.8274

[116] Daliri S, Boujarfi S, El Mokaddam A, Scholte Op Reimer WJM, Ter Riet G, den Haan C, et al. Medication-related interventions delivered both in hospital and following discharge: A systematic review and meta-analysis. BMJ Quality and Safety. 2021;**30**(2):146-156. DOI: 10.1136/bmjqs-2020-010927

[117] Schedlbauer A, Davies P, Fahey T. Interventions to improve adherence to lipid lowering medication. Cochrane Database of Systematic Reviews. 2010;(3):Cd004371. DOI: 10.1002/14651858.CD004371.pub3

[118] Pérez-Jover V, Mira JJ, Carratala-Munuera C, Gil-Guillen VF, Basora J, López-Pineda A, et al. Inappropriate use of medication by elderly, polymedicated, or multipathological patients with chronic diseases. International Journal of Environmental Research and Public Health. 2018;**15**(2):1-14. DOI: 10.3390/ijerph15020310

[119] Prakasam D, Wong AL, Smithburger PL, Buckley MS, Kane-Gill SL. Benefits of patient/caregiver engagement in adverse drug reaction reporting compared with other sources of reporting in the inpatient setting: A systematic review. Journal of Patient Safety. 2021;**17**(8):e765-ee72. DOI: 10.1097/pts.0000000000000734

[120] Hailu GN, Abdelkader M, Asfaw F, Meles HA. Exploring the knowledge and skills for effective family caregiving in elderly home care: A qualitative study. BMC Geriatrics. 2024;**24**(1):342. DOI: 10.1186/s12877-024-04924-3

[121] Mthembu TG, Brown Z, Cupido A, Razack G, Wassung D. Family caregivers' perceptions and experiences regarding caring for older adults with chronic diseases. South African Journal of Occupational Therapy. 2016;**46**(1):83-88. DOI: 10.17159/2310-3833/2016/v46n1a15